Praise for *The Herbal Epicure*

"This highly intriguing and appealing book will be very useful for anyone with both a kitchen and an herb garden."

—ANNEMARIE COLBIN
Author of *Food and Healing*
and *Food and Our Bones*

"*The Herbal Epicure* will inspire you to get right out in your garden, harvesting and creatively preparing healthful and delicious foods. Carole Ottesen's talent as both a gardener and a cook . . . are phenomenal. I am thrilled to have so many new recipes to bring into my own kitchen."

—HOLLY H. SHIMIZU
Managing Director
Lewis Ginter Botanical Garden

"Carole Ottesen has produced an encyclopedic volume which should be a cornerstone in every gardener's bookshelf. A brilliant book, well illustrated, clearly written, and copiously annotated. For all of those questions you had on herbs, their growing, harvesting, and culinary uses, this is a one-stop information center."

—HOWARD-YANA SHAPIRO, PH.D.
Vice President of Agriculture Seeds of Change
Author of *Gardening for the Future of the Earth*

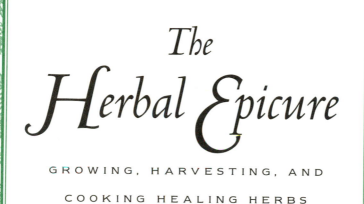

The Herbal Epicure

GROWING, HARVESTING, AND

COOKING HEALING HERBS

Carole Ottesen

Ballantine Wellspring

THE BALLANTINE PUBLISHING GROUP

NEW YORK

A Ballantine Wellspring Book
Published by The Ballantine Publishing Group
Copyright © 2001 by Carole Ottesen
Foreword by James A. Duke copyright © 2001 by James A. Duke
Foreword by James Adams copyright © 2001 by James Adams

Ballantine is a registered trademark and Ballantine Wellspring and the Ballantine
Wellspring colophon are trademarks of Random House, Inc.

www.randomhouse.com/BB/

Library of Congress Catalog Card Number: 00-110077

ISBN 0-345-43402-1

Cover design by Barbara Leff
Cover photo by Vittorio Sartor

Manufactured in the United States of America

First Edition: February 2001

10 9 8 7 6 5 4 3 2 1

Contents

Foreword by James A. Duke   xiii

Foreword by James Adams   xv

Introduction   xvii
    The Healing Garden   xvii
    The Healing Kitchen   xxii

Healing Plants for Use or for Delight   1

Aloe   3
    Using Aloe   4

Anise   5
    Aniseed Bread   7
    Anise Biscotti   7

Asparagus   9
    Sue Watterson's Asparagus and Ham Strudel   11
    Asparagus with Spring Greens   12

Bay   13
    Hopping John Cassoulet   14
    How to Make a Bouquet Garni   15

Bee Balm   17
    Monarda Vinaigrette   19
    Pasta with Bee Balm–Basil Pesto   19
    Crab Cakes with Bee Balm   20

Blueberry   22
    Russian Blueberry and Raspberry Pudding Nora   24

Broccoli   25
   Growing Sprouts   27
   Marinated Broccoli   28
   Sue Watterson's Dim Sum Broccoli   28

Burdock   30
   Burdock Soup   32

Burnet   33
   Soothing Burnet Wash   35
   Burnet Vinegar   35

Caraway   36
   Preparing Caraway Seeds for Culinary Use   37
   Caraway Crackers   38
   The Thyme Garden's Harissa   39

Carrot   40
   Carrots with Rosemary Butter   42
   A. Brockie Stevenson's Dilled, Chilled Carrot Soup   42

Chamomile   44
   Harvesting Chamomile Flowers for Tea   46
   Sleep Tea   47
   Chamomile Under-Eye Oil   47

Chaste Tree   49
   Hormone-Balance Tincture   51

Chervil   52
   Fines Herbes Oil   53

Chive   54
   Chive Vinaigrette   55
   Salmon "Scallopini" with Chive Cream   56

Cilantro, Coriander   57
   Curry in a Hurry   58
   Curried Lentils   59
   Black Bean–Cornmeal Muffins with Cilantro   60

Dandelion 62
Dandelion Root Tea 64
Dandelion Lasagna with Shiitakes 64
How to Roast Dandelion Roots 65
Jan Midgley's Classic Greens 66

Dill 68
Mrs. Adams's Salt Method for Preserving Dill 69
Tomato, Red Onion, and Dill Salad Bella Luna 70
Dill Hummus 70

Echinacea 72
Preparing Echinacea Roots for Storage 74
Echinacea Root Tea 74

Elderberry 75
Elderberry Cordial (Nonalcoholic) 76
Drying Elderberry Flowers 77
Elderberry Flowers Tempura 77

Elecampane 79
Elecampane Cordial 80

Epazote 82
Juan's Sopa de Albóndiga (Meatball Soup) 84
Sopa de Setas (Wild Mushroom Soup) 85
Epazote-Artemisia Room Freshener 85
Epazote Butter 86

Fava Beans 87
Nora's Fava Bean Succotash 88

Fennel 90
Herbes de Provence 93
Fennel, Orange, and Cabbage Salad 93
Terry Pogue's Fennel and Apple Salad 94

Feverfew 96
Feverfew-Cucumber Sandwich 98
Feverfew Tea 98

Garlic   99

Roasted Garlic and Eggplant Soup   103
Garlic Flower Stalks   104
Garlic Rosettes   104
Chunky Gazpacho with Lemon Balm   104
Roasted Garlic Grits   105

Ginger   107

Pommes de Marie-Eve   109
Gingered Pear Tart   110

Ginseng   111

Goldenseal   114

Gotu Kola   117

Calm and Centered Tea   118

Heartsease, Johnny-jump-up   119

Heartsease Salad   121

Horehound, White Horehound   122

Horehound Syrup   123

Hyssop   125

Hyssop Chicken for Sadnesse   126
Hyssop-Peach Tart   128

Lamb's-quarters   129

Lamb's-quarters Crêpes   130
Lamb's-quarters–Chickpea Curry   132

Lavender   133

Lavender Ice Cream   135
Lavender Crème Brûlée   136
Lavender Sugar   137
Lavender Spritzer   137

Lemon Balm   138

Bread Salad with Garden Thinnings   139
Lemon Balm Dressing   140

Lemongrass   142

Lemongrass Braid for Tea   144
Lemongrass Soup Asia Nora   144
Lemongrass Bows   145
Romy's Tom Khar   146
Red Snapper Fillet with Lemongrass   147

Lemon Verbena   148

Drying Lemon Verbena for Tea, Sachets, and Potpourri   149
Mellow Yellow Crème Brûlée   150
Lemon Verbena Sugar   151

Lovage   152

Lovage and Tomatoes   153
Cold Lovage-Potato Soup   154

Mexican Mint, Mexican Marigold   156

Mexican Mint and Watercress Butter   157
Mexican Mint Hollandaise   158
Eggs Benedict on Smoked Turkey Hash   159
Mexican Mint Picnic Chicken   159
Mexican Mint Dressing   160

Milk Thistle   161

Morning-After Milk Thistle Tonic   163

Mint   164

Forcing Mint for Winter Use   166
Jan's Peppermint Sorbet   166
Mint Iced Coffee   167
Lamb with a Peppermint Crust   168
Indiana Cold Mint Pea Salad   168

Mugwort   170

Long Creek Herbs Sleep Pillow   172

Mullein   173

Serene Slumber Tea   174

Nettle — 176
Nettle Tea — 178
Nettle-Flecked Parsnips and Turnips — 178
Nettle Fertilizer — 179
Nettle Soup — 179

Onion — 181
Curing Shallots and Onions — 183
Shallot Butter — 183

Parsley — 184
Kamut with Parsley and Onion Greens — 186
Parsley Butter — 186
François Dionot's Cold Fresh Herb Soup — 187
Joan Aghevli's Persian Rice — 188

Pepper — 190
Hot and Spicy Chicken Soup — 192
Queensdale Spicy Pepper Marinade — 193
Grilled Marinated Vegetables — 193

Pumpkin — 195
Storing Pumpkins — 196
Accidental Curried Pumpkin Soup — 196
Pumpkin Bread with Pepitas — 198

Purslane — 199
Stir-Fry Soup — 201

Rose — 202
Preparing Rose Hip Purée — 204
Rose Hip Coffee Cake — 205
Cold Season Rose Hip Chili — 206
The Only Good Fruitcake — 207
Joan's Mast-O-Khiar — 208
Rose Water — 209

Rosemary — 210
Rosemary Shortbread — 212
Mary Cooper's Rosemary Cookies — 213

Saffron   214
Using Saffron   216
Joan Aghevli's Saffron Ice Cream   216
Nora's Saffron Risotto with Shrimp and Peas   217

Sage   219
Sage Oatcakes   221
Sage Gargle   222
Sage Applesauce   222

Saint-John's-wort   223
Saint-John's-wort Oil   225

Saw Palmetto   226
Prostate-Preserving Tonic   228

Spinach   229
Shiitake Creamed Spinach   230
Spinach and Ham Strudel   231

Stevia   233
Stevia Syrup   235

Strawberry   236
Strawberry Leaf Tea   237
Sue's Strawberry Dessert Salad   238

Sumac   239
Sumac Drink and Sorbet   240

Sunflower   241
Curing Sunflower Seeds   242
Jerusalem Artichokes   243
Hunter-Gatherer Breakfast Mix   243

Thyme   245
Homemade Zahtar   246
Thyme-Ginger Dressing   247

Tomato   248
Fried Green Tomatoes à la Steve Durough   249
X's Aunt's Tomato Chutney   250

Valerian 251
Knockout Decoction 253

Lists of Healing Plants by Use 255

Sources 261

Bibliography 263

Index 267

Foreword

by James A. Duke

$\mathcal{A}$t the start of the new millennium, it is estimated that 20 percent of North Americans, largely uninsured or underinsured, will be unable to afford our hi-tech pharmaceuticals, many of which are extracted from herbs or synthesized from herbal starting materials. The United States has only recently begun to follow the lead of countries like Germany and the Caribbean countries whose governments have appointed panels of scientists to test and identify cheap, safe, and practical herbs for home use. They published their findings in modern herbals—the Commission E report from Germany and the TRAMIL Commission report from the Caribbean countries.

I propose a Commission USA, a body of distinguished scientists of many disciplines—botany, chemistry, herbalism, naturopathy, and phytochemistry—along with physicians and pharmacists. Commission USA would come together, review the data, and make suggestions and recommendations for approval of selected herbs. Most of these herbs are already widely sold here in the United States and may be safer and even more efficacious than the competing pharmaceuticals.

My friend Carole has selected and written about a number of plants with promising medicinal and outstanding nutritional properties. Beginning in the garden and moving into the kitchen, she provides sound information on how to coax them into growing for you, and then how to harvest, handle, and prepare them. The best quality of Carole's recipes is that they are mindful of health without overreminding you that they are healthful. The burdock soup recipe may well launch this "new" vegetable into haute cuisine. Some homeowners may even throw away their weed killers and dine on dandelion lawns. Eating from a healing kitchen garden may leave us thinner, the planet greener, and both healthier.

I feel blessed to find everything needed to know, grow, and make use of a great selection of healing plants, here in *The Herbal Epicure*.

James A. Duke, author of *The Green Pharmacy*

Foreword

by James Adams

*H*ardly a week goes by these days without our seeing an article or hearing a report about herbs and their healing properties. Some of the uses described are controversial and some represent accepted practice, but herbs and their healing properties have definitely caught the attention of many people. The same plants our ancestors relied upon for their medicines are being rediscovered. Herbal remedies are becoming a booming industry. What is fascinating about this trend is that many of these plants being made popular by the media are not rarities, but plants we already grow in our gardens as ornamentals.

In a public garden in Washington, D.C., I have had visitors ask to see plants of *Echinacea* that they take to help fight a cold. When I pointed out *Echinacea*, they remarked, "That's it? No, that's purple coneflower. I grow that in my garden."

People expect a plant with significant medicinal properties to be unusual, not a well-known, easily grown garden flower. The truth is that most healing herbs are not as strange and magical as we think. From angelica to violas to the dandelions that grow in our lawns, the majority are common, everyday plants.

In this book, Carole Ottesen demystifies healing herbs. She teaches us how to grow them and when and how to harvest them, and she offers many interesting—and delicious—ways to use them.

James Adams, Horticulturist

Introduction

THE HEALING GARDEN

There is life in the ground; it goes into the seeds; and it also, when it is stirred up, goes in the man who stirs it. —Charles Dudley Warner,
My Summer in a Garden, 1870

Twenty-two years ago, I moved my family to an old house in what was then still country. The house was in woeful condition—the roof leaked, some of the window frames were rotten, and there was a substantial rodent population—but the house had been a secondary consideration. The main attraction was the land: five acres, enough to allow us to become self-sufficient, to live off what I would grow in the garden and orchard.

I never did completely sever ties to the grocery store and become entirely self-sufficient. I did, however, attain another goal: I grew an abundance of excellent-tasting foods—greens, vegetables, and herbs—that brought a wonderful variety of flavors to our table. Although I had begun the food garden in a quantitative frame of mind—calculating how many rows of beans would yield enough to freeze, how many tomato plants would allow for sauce—my emphasis shifted irrevocably to quality. Eventually that quest for quality extended to food preparation as well.

You can't watch a flower become a squash and not marvel at the tremendous energy that goes into the production of a single vegetable. Sometime during a sultry day, while watering the beans or pulling out weeds, I saw a plant bear fruit and suddenly comprehended that I was observing a miracle. Witnessing that miracle turned a practical, nononsense attitude toward food into reverence.

Vegetables in their freshly harvested splendor astonished me then and still do. They are infinitely more flavorful and satisfying when taken straight out of the garden, their tastes so vivid that in the depths of winter I can salivate at the mere thought of the first delicate lettuces or a succulent garden tomato.

The superiority of homegrown produce changed the pecking order of foods on my table. Vegetables would never again serve as pallid accompaniments to a meat course. And herbs became mainstays in the kitchen.

One of my first successful garden installations had been a small plot of herbs. These highly aromatic plants didn't get eaten by deer or insects, and they grew abundantly. Gratitude may have inspired my first efforts to use them, but it wasn't long before herbal flavorings became a necessity in my cooking. Herbs also grew prolifically enough to prompt some of my first experiments with medicinal tisanes, herbal teas. Early on, I realized that these plants contained substances that worked to calm, to induce sleep, or to invigorate.

It took only one or two harvests to make me feel more that I was at the service of what the garden produced than that the garden was there to serve me. No longer did I seek the ingredients to fill recipes; rather, I sought out recipes that showcased beautiful vegetables and flavorful herbs.

As is bound to happen for anyone who establishes a kitchen garden, sheer respect for the produce carried over into the way I cooked it. Nothing short of mindful, skillful preparation would do.

Deciding that my plain, seat-of-my-pants cooking was not worthy of my materials, I began to read cookbooks, to watch cooking shows, and to experiment endlessly. I was fortunate in having cooking professionals as friends. Short stays in Africa and France and longer ones in the Cook Islands and India introduced me to new, exotic vegetables and reinforced the notion that diet is the basis of good health. Eventually I attended l'Academie de Cuisine, Washington's foremost cooking school.

Formal study of cooking gave me the confidence to experiment and create my own recipes. About half of the recipes in this book are my own, inspired by folklore or, more often, whatever was available in the garden at the time. The other half includes recipes inspired by or adapted from others, treasured recipes from friends, and outstandingly delicious ones from chefs and teachers.

Nurturing my own sustenance had not only turned me into a cook, it had made me a connoisseur. After plucking perfect greens or the plumpest beans, or waiting through the majestic ripening of a single tomato, I saw the produce in the supermarket as piles of lifeless things. Bloodless and dull, they had no tie to the taut, tangy vegetables and fruits I had harvested.

The garden spoiled me. In the off-seasons, I found myself forever pacing the produce aisles of supermarkets, not finding what I wanted to eat there. Food that is many times removed from its source is not the same. And, often, it isn't clean. According to organic herb grower Steven Smith, "Some three hundred fifty active pesticide ingredients are allowed for use on food crops—at least seventy of which have been classified by the EPA as probable or possible human carcinogens."

The surest way to have produce that hadn't been exposed to industrial toxins, I reasoned, was to grow your own in your own organic garden. That way you would know that it was clean and pure. With that, I became an organic gardener, something that sounds a lot more impressive and labor intensive than it is. I have found that with a thorough preparation of the soil and consistent watering, organic gardening actually takes less effort than conventional gardening methods, because you aren't forever spraying plants and getting worked up over bugs.

As gardening became an integral part of my life, something else happened. At first I couldn't put my finger on it. I suspected that, wonderful though they were, healthful food and flavorings were not the sum total of the garden's blessings. Then one day I stormed into the garden after a particularly vexing day. Almost instantly I calmed down. It was then I realized that I had a decompression/detoxification chamber just outside the door: the garden.

In doing the work of the garden—the bending, lifting, digging, walking, carrying—I exercised with a purpose seldom encountered in other parts of life. And while I worked, the stresses heaped upon me in all of the other roles I assumed in a complex life fell away.

It's no longer news that exercise and good health are linked. Everybody knows it. The studies undertaken on exercise and how it influences our state of health are legion. What isn't as obvious is that you don't have to do exercise with a big "E." You don't have to take a class or buy a rowing machine or squeeze into a leotard or invest in a mountain bike to keep fit.

Working in the garden will do the job gently but thoroughly. Gardening is weight-bearing work that stretches and tones and is sometimes aerobic. It brings on the "good" kind of tiredness and the deep, sound sleep remembered from childhood. Experts estimate that a 140-pound woman gardening burns about 315 calories each hour—about the same amount as would be expended in low-impact aerobics. A garden can be your personal fitness machine.

The beauty of gardening is that when you are doing it, you don't find yourself looking at the clock and waiting for it to be over. Instead, hours may pass before you notice the sun getting low on the horizon and a great weariness overtaking you. You have spent far longer than anticipated because you lost yourself in your tasks. When that happened, you were engaged in vigorous meditation.

While you shovel the compost, tie up the tomatoes, or dig pokeweed from the fava beans, you enter that stressless state in which mind and body are in balance. If there were instruments hooked up to you to measure blood pressure, heart rate, and other indicators of your state of being, they would agree: gardening calms both mind and body.

Some people react as predictably as Pavlov's dog, having only to walk into the garden to feel stress fall away.

We've known that "stress kills" for a long time. Now, medical scientists are finding more subtle patterns between personality, behavior, and illness. Jon Kabat-Zinn, director of the Stress Reduction Clinic at the University of Massachusetts Medical Center, notes: "As we begin looking at chronic illnesses like cancer and heart disease, which aren't infectious, we see more and more evidence that how we live our lives and, in fact, how we think and feel over a lifetime can influence the kinds of illnesses that we have."

The connection between health and state of mind is not only powerful, new research suggests it may be highly specific. Type A personalities, for example, have been known to suffer a greater incidence of cardiovascular illness. John E. Sarno, M.D., the author of *Healing Back Pain: The Mind-Body Connection*, notes that people with conscientious perfectionist personalities often suffer from fibromyalgia. Now scientists are investigating possible links between various cancers and personality types.

According to Christiane Northrup, M.D., author of *Women's Bodies,*

Women's Wisdom, "Every thought, every emotion is a biochemical reaction in your body." The body is a mirror of the mind. The thinking brain can actually stimulate the manufacture of white cells that boost immunity. Or, as in experiments conducted by Dr. Candace Pert, stress can lower white blood cell count, making a person more susceptible to illness.

People who enjoy good health are positive in their thinking and have peace of mind. The kinds of calm, positive thoughts generated by working in a garden create a healing state of mind.

An added boon to garden work is that just being outside in the fresh air links people to their environment. You can't establish a healing kitchen garden without hitching yourself to the rhythms of nature, to sun, rain, and temperature. Caught up in the cycle of the seasons, watching dry seeds spring to life in spring and plants flourishing in the summer, you live in harmony with the earth.

There is a silent dialogue between people and nature. When it is harmonious, it becomes positive and supportive. From this harmony comes profound psychic and physical comfort.

Sitting at a desk or at the wheel in the car, standing behind a counter, you may be unaware that you even have a nose. When you garden, you're as conscious of scent as any dog. You can sense a spring thaw coming by the aroma of the breathing earth. You can smell summer rain in the next county. You can smell your way through the herb garden blindfolded.

The world outside the garden may be out of control, but inside the garden walls you exercise enormous influence over your own small piece of earth. You can't heal the environment, but you can make your garden the way the rest of the world ought to be. You can heal your own small sphere and leave no room for poisons—chemicals or thoughts. That is a small but certain step toward an environmentally sound planet.

An organic garden is a good model for understanding how maintaining health through balance works. All organic gardeners provide optimum conditions for their plants to make them strong. Grown without stress, with adequate nutrition and micronutrients, enough water, the preferred amount of light, and good air circulation, these plants stay healthy. They don't succumb to serious illness and they withstand insect attack without chemicals. The same is true for other living things, including ourselves.

Health, like a good investment, is steadily, quietly cumulative. It isn't the result of a dose of miracle vitamins or a magic-bullet drug. Rather, maximizing physical well-being is an ongoing process that involves unpolluted nutrition, micronutrients, water, and air. Because people are beings that move and think, exercise and spiritual nourishment are crucial components. By systematically providing these things for ourselves, we can achieve the state of physical and mental balance that is glowing good health.

THE HEALING KITCHEN

But right now, we can't understand which phytochemicals prevent which cancers, so we can't put them in a pill. And even when we do understand, the simplest recommendation is still going to be to eat vegetables and fruit.
—John D. Potter, Head of Cancer Prevention and Research
    at the Fred Hutchinson Cancer Research Center in Seattle,
    Washington, and Professor of Epidemiology at the University of
    Washington School of Public Health and Community Medicine

"You are what you eat" is a notion that's been around for a long time. It was the sort of thing your grandmother said, not your doctor. Until recently, questions about diet were not a part of a routine medical exam. The connection between food and health was somehow too vague to be scientific.

Now that is changing. New research into how the compounds in food plants affect people is burgeoning. Each new study of these phytochemicals adds another piece to the puzzle of how we stay healthy and why we get ill. The big picture that is emerging shows that what we eat can help prevent and cure disease.

For optimal health, we may have to change what we eat. It seems simple. Eat the good stuff, exercise, and rest and you'll live a long, healthy life. Beta-carotene is good, right? You need vitamin C, right? So you buy some beta-carotene pills and some vitamin C and take those, along with some flax pills for fiber, some ginseng pills for energy, some gotu kola for enhanced brain function, Saint-John's-wort for anxiety . . . and before you know it, you need three glasses of orange juice in the morning to get it all down.

Something about the quick fix of a pill is both alluringly convenient and terribly suspect. While you pop more pills than you have ever done in your life, there is, in the back of your mind, a nagging suspicion that it is too good to be true. And it is.

No amount of herbal supplements will make up for a bad diet. Absolutely nothing beats eating good food, day after day, year after year. Plant scientists who investigate phytochemicals frequently speak of "synergy"—the combined action of all the compounds in a plant, often yielding a result greater than the sum of the parts. For example, beta-carotene is a powerful antioxidant found in, among other plants, carrots. It is not the only health-enhancing substance found in carrots. In addition to beta-carotene, carrots contain vitamin C and vitamin E and vitamin A and carotenoids (of which beta-carotene is only one) and fiber. You can take all of these in the form of supplements, but they still won't add up to what you'll get from actually eating carrots.

Nutritional supplements in the form of pills or tinctures are great if there is no other way to acquire a particular nutrient or if your need for that nutrient is greater than the amount you can reasonably consume in vegetable form. In most cases, however, it's better—and infinitely more pleasant—just to eat your carrots. And your spinach. And your broccoli.

Carrots, spinach, and broccoli are three of the select group of vegetables included in this book. Unlike many herbals—exhaustive compilations of every herb used medicinally—this book features only a small group of vegetables and herbs, chosen because they met certain criteria.

First of all, these plants are worth the effort of growing them. They are amazingly nutritious or contain health-promoting compounds or both. Many of them are the sources of the supplements you can buy in health food stores.

Second, they taste good and are useful in the kitchen. Some of them are hybrids, especially bred for taste or to contain higher amounts of specific compounds than ordinary varieties.

Third, the plants in this book were chosen because they are safe. Plants such as angelica or borage with long histories of medicinal use had to be omitted because they are suspected of containing possible carcinogens.

Finally, these plants are growable. No matter where you live—even if it's in an apartment—you can grow some of them.

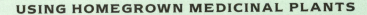
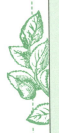

USING HOMEGROWN MEDICINAL PLANTS

Growing your own medicinal plants will demystify them. It is amazingly simple to grow the things that you see dried and powdered in capsules or distilled in tinctures. The advantage to growing your own is that you know your product is organic, pure, and clean. But there is a disadvantage: the dosage is not standardized.

For this reason, of all the hundreds of herbs, the ones in this book are a small, select collection, chosen for absolute safety. And the safest and easiest way to use your homegrown herbs is in teas or decoctions.

Teas are made from the fresh or dried leaves of plants steeped in water that has been heated to boiling. Unless otherwise specified, a general rule is to use about one heaping tablespoon of dried leaves or a half cup of fresh ones to eight ounces of water.

Decoctions are made from sterner stuff: twigs or bark or hard seeds. These materials don't release their essences with mere steeping; they require ten to twenty minutes of simmering to yield a tea-like drink. Both teas and decoctions are strained before drinking. Generally, no more than three cups of tea or decoction are drunk daily.

Even when tightly sealed, dried herbs begin to lose their essence after three months. For longer preservation, you can make a tincture, the essence of the herb infused in alcohol. Tinctures last up to three years.

Unless otherwise specified, the general rule for making tinctures is to combine one part of the herb to ten parts of pure grain alcohol in a jar. The herbs are completely covered with the alcohol. The jar is covered and the contents are shaken daily for two weeks. Then the liquid is filtered and the tincture bottled. Thirty drops of tincture is a typical dose.

A few points to keep in mind:

- Make sure a plant is what you think it is. Patronize reputable nurseries and keep careful records of plants you start from seed.
- If you are pregnant, be wary of any herb and avoid taking medicinal quantities (more than ordinary culinary quantities).
- Start slowly with any herb. You might be allergic. Anyway, if a little bit is good, more may not be.
- Don't ingest herbs that are moldy or appear diseased (a bug bite or two is fine).

The action of a good diet and herbs is slow, but the rewards are great. Be patient.

Your own garden is your best possible source of healthful foods. Perhaps its greatest advantage is that it allows you to custom-design a diet based on your own nutritional and medical needs. You can grow a perennial border of plants to cure colds and flu. You can design a tea garden. You can landscape with plants to support your prostate gland or prevent PMS. You can plant blood-purifying herbs for beautiful skin.

Once you've coaxed vegetables and herbs out of the earth, you're halfway there. The final leg of the journey is the crucial passage from garden to table.

There is an unfortunate association between good-for-you food and bland taste. Resigning ourselves to boring food in the name of health is a joyless, soul-shriveling attitude that cannot possibly be good for us. Food can best heal the body when it delights the palate.

As the fruits of your garden pass through your kitchen, celebrate them and prepare them in ways that lift the spirit—even if it takes a little butter or cream. I have made a choice in my own kitchen to cook with the finest ingredients in the most tasteful way. The ingredients may include meats, cream, butter, cheeses, and nuts. These foods are often also an efficient means of obtaining essential nutrients. By limiting the amounts of these sometimes high-calorie foods to small, sensible portions, you can satisfy your senses and appetite and probably curb the odd craving for junk foods, too.

When cooking from the garden, you must respond to both the glut and the dearth of harvest, so it is always a creative challenge. Experiment freely. Some of the recipes in this book—Dill Hummus, Chunky Gazpacho with Lemon Balm, Mellow Yellow Crème Brûlée—came about from dealing with "freaks of harvest." Most recipes can be pleasantly altered by the addition of an herb or green or vegetable. If all else fails, make soup and enjoy the preparation.

No matter what you make, you will feel enormous satisfaction in working with produce that you have nurtured. You will find that cooking centers the mind through activity. In the midst of your obligations and responsibilities, cooking can be the calming pause that gently gathers up flying thoughts and brings attention to the here and now. After a tense day, it is infinitely soothing to allow the hands to busy themselves in rituals of preparation as thoughts slow down and center inward.

All cooking connects people to their food. When you prepare food that you have grown yourself, you connect to the earth and share that connection with all who partake of the meal. To paraphrase the prophet, cooking is love made edible.

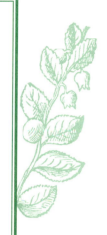

Healing Plants for Use or for Delight

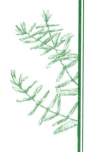

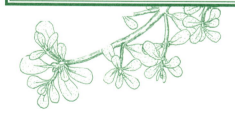

Aloe

BOTANICAL NAME: *Aloe vera,* Liliaceae.

COMMON NAME: Aloe.

DESCRIPTION: Perennial, evergreen succulent.

> *Height:* To 2 feet.

> *Flowers:* Yellow, on long stems.

> *Leaves:* Fleshy, pale green, sometimes spotted white, with spines.

HARVEST: Cut leaves for gel as needed.

CULTURE: Zones 9 and 10. Aloe will live contentedly in a container, requires fast-draining soil, and will survive in light shade.

USE: Gel from aloe leaves is soothing for burns, psoriasis, and itchy scalp.

COMMENTS: When taken internally, aloe gel is a dangerously potent purgative.

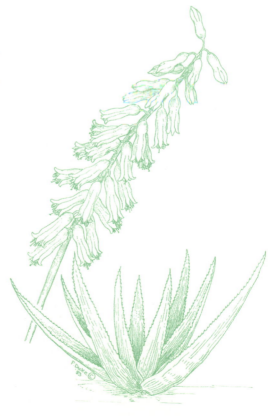

Nearly thirty years ago, I bought an aloe plant at a roadside stand in Florida. Despite benign neglect, that plant grew into a great strapping specimen, eventually producing a necklace of young plants at its base. Then, one fatal fall, I left the aloe family outside too long. The mother plant froze and seemed to melt away, but in the shelter of the big plant some of the babies survived—including one that lives in my sunniest window today. Aloe is an easy-to-grow, forgiving plant.

Aloe has been used medicinally since pharaonic times to treat burns, to reduce excess mucus, and to embalm. It is said that Cleopatra was massaged with aloe gel to make her skin beautiful. Later, Pliny, the Roman naturalist, recommended that aloe be taken internally as a laxative. Modern scientific studies show that these traditional uses are valid. According to Dr. James Duke's database, aloe gel is anti-inflammatory and antiseptic, and is a moisturizer and a tissue restorative. It is safe and effective for external use.

Aloe is superb for burns, itching, and sunburn and has been used to treat radiation burns. The leaves contain a clear gel that is tremendously soothing and speeds healing. When the gel dries, it forms a natural, see-through bandage. Mixed with almond, olive, or coconut oil, the gel is effective in healing psoriasis.

The German Commission E placed aloe on its approved list as effective for constipation. However, taken internally, aloe is a powerful purgative; it is all too easy to overdose. I strongly recommend you stick to external applications with this plant.

Using Aloe

1. Cut an outer leaf from the base of the plant.
2. With a sharp knife, make a slit on the flat side of the leaf from the base to the tip. Be careful not to cut all the way through.
3. Fold back the outer skin of the leaf to expose the inside.
4. Scrape out the gel with a spoon.
5. Apply the gel to burned skin, mix it into shampoo, or add it to suntan lotion.

Anise

PIMPINELLA ANISUM

BOTANICAL NAME: *Pimpinella anisum,* Apiaceae.

COMMON NAME: Anise.

DESCRIPTION: Annual.

> *Height:* To 2 feet.
>
> *Flowers:* White umbels like those of Queen Anne's lace in summer.
>
> *Leaves:* Licorice-scented on lax stems; they are toothed at the base of the plant and change, as they move up the stem, to lacy at the top.

HARVEST: Snip leaves and flowers for salads; cut umbels of seeds as soon as they begin to turn tan.

CULTURE: Sow seeds in light, well-drained soil of low fertility or start indoors in deep peat pots.

USE: Seeds are a digestive, effective for flatulence, and have estrogenic activity; they may be useful for symptoms of menopause; the leaves spice salads.

COMMENTS: To harvest seeds for personal use, you'll need at least six plants for cooking, more if you wish to use the seeds for tea.

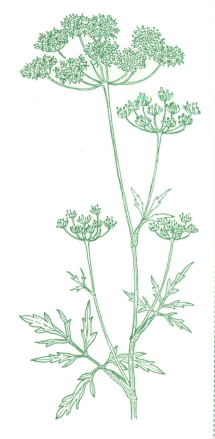

*A*nise provides leaves for tasty additions to salads and licorice-tasting seeds for flavoring curries, cookies, cakes, and bread. An annual plant that reaches just over a foot tall, tap-rooted anise grows best when sown directly in the garden in a sunny, well-drained place. Like basil, anise grows faster when the weather gets hot.

Leaves may be harvested at any time. The seeds follow flowers that look like tiny Queen Anne's lace (both plants are members of the carrot family) and don't mature until late summer or early fall. The flowers as well as the leaves are good in salad.

Though anise is considered primarily a flavoring in this country, in other parts of the world it is highly respected as a digestive, a fungicide, and an expectorant. It has been a part of traditional remedies for centuries. Chinese, Ayurvedic, and early European herbalists esteemed anise as a digestive, very effective for flatulence. No less a physician than Hippocrates prescribed anise as a remedy for clearing the respiratory system; it has been used for coughs and bronchitis ever since. The German Commission E approved anise for catarrh and dyspeptic conditions.

Research affirms that anise contains anethole, a compound similar in its effects to estrogen. This is likely the basis for its traditional use as an aphrodisiac and the reason that anise may help reduce menopausal symptoms. It may also serve as part of a plant-based hormone therapy.

A nice way to make use of anise's digestive properties is to bake it into biscotti to be enjoyed after dinner with a healing tea. Or bake aniseed into an unusual and delicious bread.

Anise is an annual, best started indoors in peat pellets to minimize transplant shock. It will reach a height of two feet in rather rich but well-drained soil in full sun or very light shade.

The seed, renowned for flavoring anisette and Pernod, is the most medicinally active part of the plant. Each plant produces only a scant teaspoonful of seed. For a winter's worth of tea, you'll need several dozen plants and you'll have to refrain from cutting too many of the flowers for salads. Anise's stems and roots will add a hint of licorice to soups.

Aniseed Bread

Aniseed lends a gentle and unexpected licorice flavor that makes this bread almost addictive. You can also add anise seeds to your own favorite bread recipe.

3 ⅓ cups all-purpose flour
  2 teaspoons salt
  1 package active dry yeast
  1 tablespoon sugar
1 ¼ cups milk
  1 egg
  2 teaspoons aniseed

1. Preheat the oven to 400°.
2. Combine the flour and salt in a mixing bowl.
3. Combine the yeast and sugar in a cup.
4. Warm the milk and add 2 tablespoons of it to the yeast mixture. Mix together and let stand for 10 minutes.
5. Beat the egg into the rest of the milk. Add the aniseed to the milk mixture.
6. Add the yeast mixture and the milk mixture to the flour and stir well.
7. When the dough holds together, knead it until it is smooth and elastic.
8. Let the dough rise in a warm place until doubled in volume. Punch down and knead for 5 minutes.
9. Place the dough in a buttered loaf pan (10 × 4 × 3 inches), put it in a warm place, and let it rise again.
10. Bake 40 to 45 minutes.

YIELD: 1 loaf, serves 6 to 8

Anise Biscotti

Sue Watterson, chef at the Café Bethesda and a popular teacher at Washington's premier cooking school, l'Academie de Cuisine, shared this recipe. She suggests using chopped figs instead of the cherries, but I'm a cherry lover.

2½ cups flour
1 cup sugar
½ teaspoon baking soda
½ teaspoon baking powder
Pinch of salt
1–2 tablespoons Pernod or any anise-flavored liqueur
1½ cups chopped dried cherries (or dried figs)
3 eggs, beaten
Zest of 1 orange
2 teaspoons aniseed, lightly toasted

1. Preheat the oven to 350°.
2. Place the flour, sugar, baking soda, baking powder, and salt in a mixing bowl. Mix briefly to combine.
3. Warm the liqueur and rehydrate the cherries in it. Add the eggs, orange zest, aniseed, and cherries to the dry ingredients, mixing just until a dough is formed.
4. Turn the dough out onto a lightly floured surface and knead briefly. Divide into 2 pieces. Working with a piece at a time, roll the dough into logs, each about 2 inches wide.
5. Place the logs on greased or parchment-lined baking sheets and flatten them slightly.
6. Bake at 350° for 15 to 20 minutes, until the logs feel set when touched. Remove them from the oven and reduce the oven temperature to 250°.
7. Let the logs become cool to the touch, then slice them into ½-inch pieces. Lay each piece on its side on the baking sheet, a cut side facing up.
8. Bake for an additional 15 to 20 minutes at 250°, or until the biscotti have dried and hardened. Alternatively, you may turn the oven off after the first bake and leave the sliced cookies on the baking sheets overnight.

YIELD: 40 biscotti

Asparagus

ASPARAGUS OFFICINALIS

BOTANICAL NAME: *Asparagus officinalis,* Liliaceae.

COMMON NAME: Asparagus.

DESCRIPTION: Deciduous perennial.

Height: To 5+ feet.

Flowers: Inconspicuous in summer.

Leaves: Feathery, bright green.

HARVEST: In spring as the shoots appear.

CULTURE: Hardy to Zone 3, asparagus needs a period of winter dormancy. Grow in a very fertile, well-prepared bed; full sun with good drainage.

USE: Asparagus is a gentle diuretic, tonic for the kidney and bowels, and vermifuge; it is a possible anticancer plant.

COMMENTS: Asparagus plants may produce edible shoots for twenty years or more.

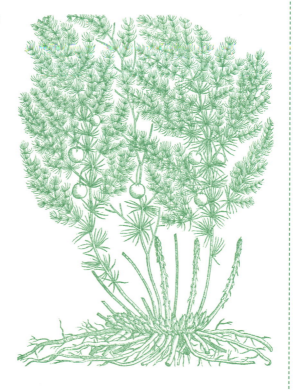

*G*rowing asparagus is a long-term garden project, but one well worth the effort of preparing the bed and waiting out the time for the plants to gain strength. The beauty of asparagus is that once they have been planted, they come up year after year, providing prized spring vegetables.

The classic method of growing asparagus is to buy two-year-old roots that look like fat gray spiders. Then you begin the arduous preparation of the bed. You dig down about twelve inches and set the roots on little mounds of soil; then you gradually refill the trenches as the plants grow. An easier method is to set the roots on soil mounds on top of the ground in what will eventually be a raised bed. Add soil between the plants, up to the top of the mounds. Then, as the plants grow, add more and more soil until the roots are a good ten to twelve inches below the surface. Use stones or boards to support the raised bed.

In the first year, the plants produce skinny little shoots. These are not to be cut, but allowed to grow and produce foliage. The following spring, the emerging shoots will be plumper—like the asparagus you see in the supermarket—and you can harvest these, but sparingly. The shoots you don't harvest will grow into tall, feathery stalks to nourish the plant for the next year's harvest.

If you start asparagus from seed instead of buying the roots, you'll have to wait until the third season to cut asparagus.

Asparagus is a perfect plant for the healing garden because it is not only a delicious specialty vegetable, but is truly healing in the most gentle way. Rich in folic acid, which is thought to prevent cervical cancer, it is also a restorative and cleansing vegetable for the bowels, the liver, and the kidneys. The German Commission E approved asparagus rhizomes for a tea to help treat inflammatory kidney disease. Asparagus contains asparagustic acid, useful in treating cystitis, pyelitis, and parasitic worms. But you don't have to think about all of that. Just enjoy asparagus and know they are good for you.

Asparagus lend themselves to dozens of cooking applications, but they are splendid when served simply with butter, salt, and pepper. Or try them with Mexican Mint Hollandaise (page 158).

Sue Watterson's Asparagus and Ham Strudel

Chef Sue Watterson suggests serving this beautiful strudel for brunch. You'll get rave reviews. The only difficult part is working with the phyllo dough. Make sure it is completely defrosted before attempting to unroll it. Keep a clean, dry tea towel handy to cover the sheets you are not working with, because the dough dries out quickly (and sticks to anything wet). And remember that even if you rip the dough, you can patch the tears with the second layer.

    1 pound asparagus
    6 sheets of phyllo dough, thawed
    6 ounces (12 tablespoons) butter, clarified
    1 egg white, lightly beaten
    6 ounces Gruyère, grated
    ½ pound ham, thinly sliced

1. Preheat the oven to 375°.
2. Trim off and discard the tough stem ends of the asparagus. Blanch the stalks in boiling salted water until just tender, 5 to 8 minutes. Refresh under cold water, drain, and pat dry. Set aside.
3. Place one sheet of phyllo dough, long side toward you, on a clean, flat work surface. Brush with clarified butter.
4. Place a second sheet on top of the first; brush the surface of the second sheet with butter. Repeat until you have a stack of five sheets.
5. Lay the sixth sheet on top of the others; brush the surface of this last sheet with some of the beaten egg white.
6. Sprinkle the grated cheese over the last phyllo layer, leaving a 2-inch border of dough on each side.
7. Place the slices of ham, overlapping slightly, on top of the cheese in a single layer. Place the asparagus lengthwise in three columns, tips all pointing the same way, on top of the ham. The asparagus stalks should be lined up next to one another in each column.
8. Starting with the long end of the phyllo nearest you, start rolling the stacked sheets of dough around the filling. Roll gently but

firmly in jelly roll fashion, until the filling is completely wrapped and you have a stuffed tube of dough. This is your strudel.

9. Carefully place the strudel on a lightly greased or parchment-lined baking sheet and brush the outside surface of the strudel with the remaining egg white.

10. Bake for 20 to 25 minutes, or until the strudel is crisp and browned. Let stand for 5 minutes before slicing.

YIELD: 4 to 6 servings

Asparagus with Spring Greens

On the morning of a spring dinner party, I get out in the garden early to pick lettuces and asparagus. A typical mixture might include Black-Seeded Simpson lettuce, burnet, tat soi, mâche, spinach, violet leaves, sorrel, and garlic and onion greens. These are washed, spun dry, and then crisped in linen towels encased in plastic bags in the refrigerator. Later on, they are arranged on salad plates with the cooled, cooked asparagus. Each plate is then covered with plastic wrap and stored in the refrigerator. The dressing goes on just before this quick and easy first course is served.

8 asparagus
1 quart bowl of salad greens, washed, dried, and crisped
　　Colorful component: Johnny-jump-ups, violet flowers, rose petals
　　Lemon Balm Dressing (page 140)

1. Cook the asparagus in boiling, salted water until they are bright green. Plunge into ice water and cool.

2. Arrange the salad greens, asparagus, and rose petals or a flower or two on four salad plates. Cover with plastic wrap until ready to serve.

3. Unwrap each plate carefully to avoid disturbing the arrangement and drizzle 2 to 3 teaspoons of Lemon Balm Dressing over each salad.

YIELD: 4 servings

Bay

BOTANICAL NAME: *Laurus nobilis,* Lauraceae.

COMMON NAMES: Bay, sweet bay.

DESCRIPTION: Evergreen tree.

> *Height:* Outdoors to 30 feet; in containers, usually about 6 feet.

> *Flowers:* Small yellow flowers in summer.

> *Leaves:* Leathery, elliptical, 1 to 3 inches long.

HARVEST: As needed, or when pruning.

CULTURE: In Zone 7 and below, grow bay outside in fertile, well-drained soil in light shade; in colder climates, grow it in a container and bring it inside over winter.

USE: Bay is an important seasoning that is also a gentle digestive.

COMMENTS: Bay's flavor is more intense in dried leaves. Remove the inedible leaves from food before serving.

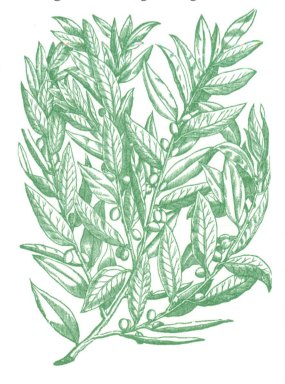

*L*ucky are those who live far enough south (or west) to be able to grow bay outside as a tree. Where winter temperatures fall below 15 degrees Fahrenheit, this tender Mediterranean native has to be potted up—ordinary potting soil will do—and brought inside to a sunny window. If your garden is right on the hardiness line for bay, a position against a wall with a southeast exposure and protection from wind and the hot afternoon sun is perfect.

Whether your bay tree grows inside or out, having one nearby means an endless supply of fresh, flavorful, leathery bay leaves. You can snip them when they are fresh off the tree, or dry them first; drying intensifies the fragrance. Some people trim bay trees into formal shapes and reserve the clippings for seasoning. Dried and stored away from heat and light, bay leaves will keep for about a year.

Especially when grown indoors, bay sometimes suffers an infestation of scale insects. These are hard-to-see, smooth, tan-colored ovals along the veins of the leaves. If you notice shiny, sticky drops of oil on the leaves, chances are your plant has scale. It is easy to control if you keep at it. Take cotton pads dipped in alcohol and clean both sides of the leaves. If possible, let the plant live outside over the summer; humidity and the presence of insect predators will help control the scale.

While not a heavy hitter medicinally, bay is an appetite stimulant and is helpful for colic and flatulence. You can make a tea from bay leaves, but by far the more delicious way to enjoy bay is to use the leaves to season soups and stews. Bay leaves are too tough to eat. Be sure to remove them from food before serving.

Bay is an essential ingredient in poaching fish and in making soups, marinades, and the classic bouquet garni.

Hopping John Cassoulet

Bay joins rosemary, whose compounds enhance brain function, and heal-all garlic and onions to be slowly baked with chicken, sausage, black-eyed peas, wine, and rice. This recipe is inspired by a black bean cassoulet published in one of the first cookbooks I ever owned, Twelve Company Dinners, *by Margo Rieman. What I learned from that recipe is that the secret to cassoulet is in the very slow cooking.*

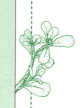

HOW TO MAKE A BOUQUET GARNI

On a 4×4-inch piece of cheesecloth, lay:

> 4 sprigs chives
> 3 sprigs parsley (or chervil)
> 2 sprigs thyme
> 1 bay leaf

Make a little hobo bag out of the cheesecloth with the herbs inside. Using 6 to 8 inches of string, tie the bundle together. Leave the string long to make it easier to pull the bouquet garni out of the pot before serving the dish.

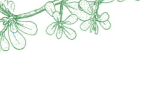

Don't take any shortcuts with this one. Bay and plentiful rosemary season chicken that is cooked to tender perfection. The black-eyed peas bring good luck when this dish is served on New Year's Day.

> 1 pound Italian sausage
> 1 chicken (3–4 pounds), skinned and cut into serving pieces, salted and peppered
> 3 onions, chopped
> 6 cloves garlic, chopped
> 3 cups red wine
> 1 can tomato sauce (8 ounces)
> 2 sprigs of rosemary (4-inch), or 1 teaspoon dried rosemary leaves
> 4 bay leaves
> 1 tablespoon dried oregano
>   Pinch of cayenne, or 1 very small, very hot chili, crushed
> 1 cup basmati or Texmati rice or kamut
> 2 cups black-eyed peas, either fresh or presoaked
> 1–2 cups bread crumbs

1. Prick and brown the sausage in a deep pan; set aside. Pour off some of the fat and brown the chicken in the same pan; set aside.
2. Cook the onions and garlic until soft, then add the sausage, chicken, wine, tomato sauce, herbs, and cayenne.
3. Simmer, covered, over very low heat, for 1 hour.
4. Preheat the oven to 200°.
5. In an ovenproof casserole with a cover, combine the rice and beans.
6. Add the pieces of sausage and chicken, deboning as you go, to the casserole. Then pour the pan juices over the rice mixture. Top with the bread crumbs.
7. Bake, covered, for 2 to 3 hours or until the rice is cooked.

YIELD: Serves 6 very hungry people

TIP

Bay has been used for centuries as a deterrent to weevils. Place 3 to 4 bay leaves in a container with flour or figs. Or add some to boxes of cereal and cornmeal to deter cereal moths.

Store bay leaves with your rice to add flavor.

Bee Balm

MONARDA DIDYMA

BOTANICAL NAME: *Monarda didyma,* Lamiaceae.

COMMON NAMES: Bee balm, Oswego tea, bergamot horsebalm.

DESCRIPTION: Deciduous perennial.

Height: 3 to 4 feet.

Flowers: Scarlet, but also white or fuchsia; in summer.

Leaves: Aromatic, medium green, on square stems.

Habit: Upright clumps spread quickly.

HARVEST: As needed.

CULTURE: Zones 4 to 9. Bee balm grows best in full to part sun with moist soil. It is a good companion to tomatoes.

USE: According to Dr. James Duke's database, monardas contain two compounds, carvacrol and thymol, which help prevent the breakdown of acetylcholine.

COMMENTS: Edible flowers. Monardas are hard-to-beat garden plants— beautiful, edible, and medicinal.

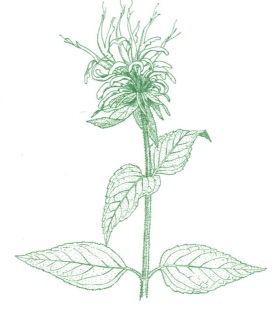

OTHER SPECIES:

Wild bergamot *(Monarda fistulosa)*; lemon bergamot *(M. citriodora)*; oregano de la sierra *(M. menthifolia).*

Oswego Indians were brewing soothing "Oswego tea" from monarda's flowers and leaves long before the first white settlers arrived in North America. While there are still pockets of intractable Oswego tea drinkers, over the centuries *Monarda didyma* came to be known primarily as an ornamental garden plant. There's a good reason for this.

If you have ever taken a hike in the woods and come upon a crowd of blooming bee balm—growing wild and shaggy and glowing a riveting crimson in a world of greens—you'll understand this plant's popularity in the garden. Gay, vivid bee balm quickly caught the attention of plant breeders, who developed cultivars such as the classic "Cambridge Scarlet" and, more recently, bold "Jacob Cline" and the mildew-resistant "Marshall's Delight" with glowing fuchsia flowers.

The place where a plant grows in the wild is always a good guide to its placement in the garden. This square-stemmed member of the mint family is at its vigorous best in rich, moist soil in a partly shaded place—the same conditions encountered in clearings or at the edge of woodland. Where conditions are favorable, it will grow to three feet or more and spread into cheerful colonies. When the central part of bee balm's root dies out—every three years or so—it is time to divide and replant the divisions.

Bee balm's relatives are also both attractive and useful. All were part of the pharmacology of Native Americans. Wild bergamot *(M. fistulosa)*, hardy from Zone 3 to Zone 10, has fuchsia-colored flowers and reaches two and a half feet tall. Annual lemon bergamot *(M. citriodora)* grows to two feet in sun or part shade. Use the fresh or dried leaves in fruit desserts and teas. The curious flowers are wonderful for bouquets. Oregano de la sierra *(M. menthifolia)* is a tall perennial, used in the Southwest to flavor wild game and ricotta cheese. Its flowers have a hot flavor and are sometimes added to salsa or chili dishes.

Given optimal conditions, monardas will spread like mint, but, like mint, they are truly tough plants and persist in lesser situations. With enough water, they'll even grow in containers. The new, purple-flowered "Petite Delight," which reaches only about a foot in height, would be ideal (when well watered) in a pot.

Having bee balm in the garden is a beautiful way to enjoy other good-for-you plants. Sprinkle scarlet bee balm petals over salad greens like confetti. Or enliven salads with lemon bergamot's exotic flowers. While you eat the flowers or drink a tea from the peppery leaves, monarda's compounds work to prevent the breakdown of acetylcholine, a neurotransmitter important in cognition and reasoning. (People with Alzheimer's frequently present an acetylcholine deficiency.)

During Revolutionary times people used the leaves of bergamot in place of China tea. A delicious modern compromise employs a mixture of one teaspoon of dried China tea with three teaspoons of fresh young bergamot leaves. Pour near-boiling water over the mixture and allow it to steep for several minutes.

Monarda Vinaigrette

Monarda leaves have a peppery flavor and lend this vinaigrette a beautiful green color. You can also make this with the flower petals. The red petals turn the dressing pink, while the purple petals of "Petite Delight" tint it lavender.

½ cup olive oil
¼ cup balsamic vinegar
2 tablespoons chopped monarda leaves (6–10), or petals
¼ teaspoon Dijon mustard
1 teaspoon salt (or more to taste)

Place all the ingredients in the blender and blend for 30 seconds.

YIELD: About ¾ cup

Pasta with Bee Balm—Basil Pesto

There are no hard-and-fast rules for pesto. The only limiting factor is taste. Try using nuts instead of pine nuts, or any flavorful green instead of the traditional basil. A mixture of brain-nourishing bee balm leaves, basil, and parsley, this recipe makes more than enough pesto for one dinner. Put the rest in a jar, covering the top of the pesto with a thin layer of olive oil to prevent discoloration, and store in the refrigerator.

1 cup bee balm leaves

½ cup basil leaves

½ cup parsley leaves

2 cloves garlic

1 tablespoon lemon juice

½ cup olive oil, or slightly more to blend easily

¼ cup (about 1½ ounces) pine nuts

½ teaspoon salt

Pasta, sufficient for number of people

Grated Parmesan, up to 1 cup

1. Blend together the bee balm, basil, parsley, garlic, lemon juice, and olive oil. Start with ½ cup of olive oil and add just enough to blend freely.

2. When the mixture is well blended, add the pine nuts and salt. Set aside.

3. Cook the pasta. Reserve ½ cup of the pasta water, and drain the pasta.

4. Put about 1 tablespoon of the pesto per serving in a small bowl; add just enough of the hot pasta water to make a smooth paste.

5. Combine the pesto with the drained pasta. Toss with the Parmesan.

YIELD: Enough pesto for 12 to 14 servings

Crab Cakes with Bee Balm

Marylanders have strong opinions about crab cakes, and I am no exception. I never order them out because cooks generally take too many liberties with them and the crab cakes end up tasting like bread crumbs instead of crab. This recipe is simple, and it adds just the right zip to the dominant taste of crab.

1 pound lump crabmeat

½ teaspoon dried mustard

½ teaspoon Old Bay seasoning

2 teaspoons flour

2 teaspoons grated shallot

2 teaspoons chopped bee balm leaves

1 teaspoon chopped burnet leaves

2 tablespoons plus 1 teaspoon mayonnaise

¼ teaspoon salt (or to taste)

Pepper

Olive oil

1. Remove any shells or cartilage from the crabmeat. Combine all ingredients except the olive oil.
2. Heat the oil in a pan while forming 5 or 6 cakes. Fry the cakes about 3 minutes on each side.

YIELD: 5 to 6 servings

TIP

Toss the petals of scarlet bee balm flowers in a salad.

Blueberry

VACCINIUM SPP.

BOTANICAL NAME: *Vaccinium corymbosum,* Evicaceae.

COMMON NAMES: Blueberry, highbush blueberry.

DESCRIPTION: A deciduous, sometimes evergreen shrub.

> *Height:* To 5+ feet.

> *Flowers:* White bell-shaped flowers in spring.

> *Leaves:* Clean, rounded, elliptical leaves turn color in fall.

HARVEST: As the berries turn deep blue.

CULTURE: Moist, acid soil in sun. Plant two varieties to cross-pollinate; fertilize with cottonseed meal.

USE: Vitamin and mineral rich. Contain proanthocyanosides that protect against macular degeneration, glaucoma, cataracts. Dried blueberries are helpful for diarrhea.

COMMENTS: If birds are a real problem, use netting, scarecrows, and other anti-bird devices (fake hawks, etc.).

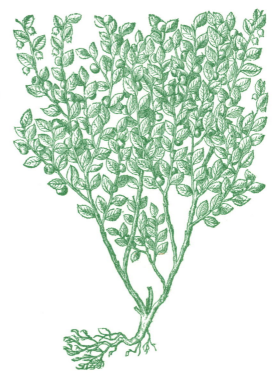

*B*lueberries were not my favorite fruit until I grew them. The difference in flavor between store-bought berries and homegrown ones is astonishing. In their first year in my garden, I ate so many right off the small, young bushes that I never really had a harvest. How nice that something so good is also good for you.

Blueberries and other berries contain plentiful fiber to aid in regularity. They are especially high in vitamins A and C and are first-rate sources of antioxidants. Like other dark fruits, they contain proanthocyanidins that help visual acuity. According to Dr. Andrew Weil, these compounds also strengthen the walls of capillaries and veins, thus helping to prevent hemorrhoids and varicose veins.

The beauty of blueberry cultivation is that it's easy—there's nothing scarily arcane about it. There's no spraying, and only the pruning out of deadwood and weak branches. If you are lucky enough to have acid soil in a sunny, moist, but well-drained place, all you do is plant the bushes and enjoy them.

The other great thing about blueberries is that the bushes are first-rate landscape plants that grow to about six feet tall. They are handsome and worthy of any spot around the house. In fall, their leaves take on vivid color.

Although there are self-fertile kinds of blueberries, such as the semi-dwarf "Sunshine Blue," it's usually best to plant two different blueberry varieties for cross-pollination. Just plant them where you can keep an eye on them in order to beat the birds to the berries.

A favorite fruit, fresh blueberries are a boon for those who suffer from urinary tract infections. Like cranberries, blueberries contain compounds that prevent bacteria from adhering to the walls of the bladder. Compounds in blueberries are also thought to help promote the production of mucus that lines the stomach.

Russian Blueberry and Raspberry Pudding Nora

This lovely dessert is quintessential Restaurant Nora, a Washington, D.C., restaurant where the freshest organic ingredients in season are served with elegant simplicity.

> 1 pint blueberries, washed and drained
> 1 pint raspberries, washed and drained
> 1 cup low-fat yogurt
> ¼ cup brown sugar
>   Mint, for garnish

1. Divide the berries among 4 individual ovenproof dishes.
2. Top each with ¼ cup of the yogurt and sprinkle with 1 tablespoon of brown sugar.
3. Broil for 3 to 5 minutes or until the sugar melts and caramelizes on the top.
4. Serve with a garnish of mint.

YIELD: 4 servings

Broccoli

BOTANICAL NAME: *Brassica oleracea* Italica Group, Cruciferae.

COMMON NAME: Broccoli.

DESCRIPTION: Annual vegetable.

   Height: To 3 feet.

   Flowers: Green, 6 to 12 inches across as terminal clusters in midsummer.

   Leaves: Wavy-edged green leaves on thick stalks.

HARVEST: Cut broccoli flowers, along with 4 to 6 inches of stem, as soon as they develop.

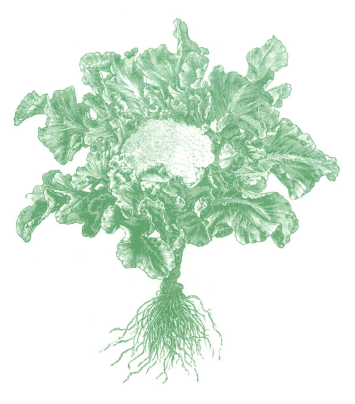

CULTURE: Plant early in spring; broccoli is tolerant of light frost and prefers cool growing conditions (below 70 degrees Fahrenheit). Give broccoli rich, deep, moist soil in full sun with good drainage; avoid sites where cabbage-family crops have previously grown.

USE: A nutritional powerhouse, broccoli is thought to help prevent cancer; it has fiber and plentiful vitamins and minerals.

COMMENTS: The richer and more evenly moist the soil, the better broccoli will tolerate the heat and the longer it will produce side shoots.

"*E*at your broccoli." We've all heard it and now we know that Mom was right. In addition to plenty of beta-carotene, broccoli contains two separate compounds that protect against cancer. And that's not all. Half a cup of broccoli will give you just about all of the vitamin C you need per day and a good part of the calcium—to say nothing of folate and fiber.

Every spring, I start broccoli plants indoors from seeds eight weeks before the last frost and transplant them into the garden at about the time of the last frost. Once the seedling is "hardened off," or acclimated to the weather outside, broccoli will not be bothered by light frosts. One of the things that make starting broccoli from seeds worth the effort is choice. Instead of the plain green, big-headed type, you can choose among Romanesco types with chartreuse heads or the purple sprouting kinds that produce multiple tender small heads.

For those who would rather not grow their own seedlings, plants of broccoli and other cabbage-family members are commonly available at garden centers as soon as it is safe to put them outdoors.

Site broccoli in rich soil in full sun. Usually, the first flower heads are ready to harvest in midsummer. They can grow as large as a foot across. Once you cut them off, the plant sends out side shoots—much smaller than the main head, but wonderful in salads. Keep cutting these off, and if the plant stays healthy you'll have an endless supply. You'll be able to eat broccoli until hard frost kills the plant.

No garden? Grow broccoli sprouts all year long on the kitchen counter. The sprouts actually contain greater concentrations of certain cancer-fighting compounds than the vegetable. Sprouts need no cooking and are great for salads or to add some crunch to sandwiches. You'll need seeds for sprouting (see Sources). These have a high germination rate and are sold in quantities suitable for sprouts. You'll also need a sprouter. Although there are specially made sprouting devices, a jar or other container that can hold water, with some sort of permeable cover, works fine.

I've used a large canning jar and placed a circle of screening (buy it at a hardware store and cut it to fit) where the removable part of the lid goes. Or you can experiment with the type of clear plastic–covered container that berries are sold in. You'll have to line the bottom with a paper towel so that the seeds don't wash away. After reading Steve Meyerowitz's *Sprouts, the Miracle Food*, I tried the willow baskets he recommends. They work extremely well as long as the basket is not too tightly woven. Baskets need routine sterilizing to deter molds.

In fact, absolute cleanliness is essential for sprout growing. The folks at Johnny's Selected Seeds, a good source of seeds to sprout, responded to the concern I expressed about *E. coli* bacteria in commercially produced sprouts with recommendations that include washing the seeds before sprouting, keeping the jar perfectly clean, refrigerating the sprouts once they are grown, and following the directions for sprouting. They also remark that broccoli as well as broccoli sprouts emit an odor, considered foul by some, that is perfectly normal.

Growing Sprouts

1. Soak seeds overnight in warm water.
2. Place them in an absolutely clean sprouter, jar, or willow basket—preferably near the sink, so you won't forget to water them.
3. Rinse the seeds thoroughly at least twice each day. If you are using a jar, fill it partly with water and shake to make sure all the seeds become wet. Then drain the water. The idea is to keep the seeds moist, but not sitting in water.
4. When the seeds begin to sprout, they will shed their shells. Wash the sprouts, allowing the shells to float away.

5. Begin to harvest sprouts when they are up and green. When they are, remove them from the sprouter and refrigerate them until ready to use. And start a new batch.

Marinated Broccoli

Bright green and tangy, broccoli marinated in Lemon Balm Dressing is a delicious vegetable for a buffet dinner. Although I love to entertain, I am one of those people who can't chew gum and walk at the same time. It helps when I can make a dish ahead of time and know that it won't lose its flavor. This one actually improves with a couple of hours in the fridge and is meant to be served cold.

Dried lemongrass leaves, optional
1 pound broccoli florets (about 3 cups)
¾ cup Lemon Balm Dressing (page 140)

1. Bring a quart of water to a boil. Add the dried lemongrass leaves, if using, to the water for flavoring.
2. Blanch broccoli for about 30 seconds, or until it is bright green.
3. Plunge the broccoli into ice water, then let it drain dry in a colander.
4. Make sure broccoli is dry. Place it in a deep bowl and pour the marinade—Lemon Balm Dressing—over it.
5. Refrigerate at least 1 hour, but don't leave it overnight. The broccoli will "cook" in the marinade. It will taste great, but it will darken.

YIELD: 4 to 6 servings

Sue Watterson's Dim Sum Broccoli

This is a great way to eat broccoli for those who—like chef Sue Watterson—really don't like it much. She writes: "You use large-ish broccoli spears, perhaps 3–4 inches long. They are meant to be grabbed with chopsticks and sorta gnawed on."

2 tablespoons cooking oil

1 tablespoon chopped ginger

8 broccoli spears (3–4 inches)

½ teaspoon soy sauce

1 teaspoon oyster sauce

1. Heat the cooking oil in a wok.
2. Toss in the chopped ginger and let sauté about 30 seconds.
3. Add the broccoli spears and stir-fry until they are bright green.
4. Add the soy sauce and oyster sauce and toss well.

YIELD: 4 servings

Burdock

ARCTIUM LAPPA

BOTANICAL NAME: *Arctium lappa,* Asteraceae.

COMMON NAME: Burdock.

DESCRIPTION: Hardy biennial.

Height: To 3 feet.

Flowers: Small, purple thistle-flowers are followed by burrs.

Leaves: Young leaves may be cooked and eaten as a green.

HARVEST: Cut young leaves; dig roots in fall of the first year or early spring of the second.

CULTURE: Zones 5 to 9; burdock has naturalized through much of the United States. In the garden, grow it in moist, loose soil in sun.

USE: Burdock is a blood purifier and immune system booster.

COMMENTS: Burdock roots are a delicious new vegetable and worth growing for their nutty flavor alone. First-year roots are carrotlike.

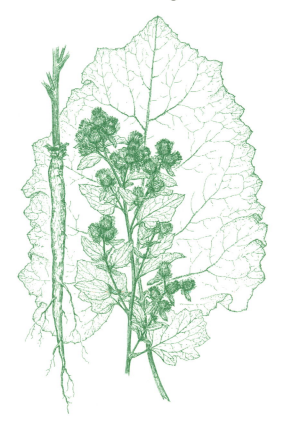

*I*t is hard to believe that the scourge of your garden is delicious stir-fried. The same weed with the sticky burrs that cling to your pants and have to be cut off your dog has roots that are called *gobo* in Japan and have been eaten as a vegetable since the tenth century.

Burdock's roots are good—*really* good—to eat and have a nutty potato flavor. And they are very, very good for you. According to Dr. James Duke's database, they are antitumor and antipyretic, and they are immunomodulators. They help in healing arthritis, lymphoma, and cystitis. When taken over longer periods of time, they have been effective in treating psoriasis and eczema. Recent research suggests that burdock may fight HIV.

Burdock is an easy-to-grow biennial, thriving even in clay soil, and producing a good-sized root after four to six months of its first season from seed, planted in spring. The root may grow to two feet long or more, but should be harvested after the first growing season. After that, all of its strength will go into production of the second year's flowering, after which the plant dies.

Because the root is long, loose soil promotes straighter roots and makes for much easier harvesting. In Japan, farmers build special boxes with high walls for growing burdock. When harvesting, the boxes are dismantled and the entire root is freed without any breakage. Such a box or some other helpful device—perhaps one of those snap-together, round compost-making bins—is necessary to procure great, long, beautiful roots that make it through the harvest in one piece. Even if you wait until after one of the first deep, penetrating rains of fall before digging, it is unlikely that you'll unearth a burdock root without leaving a piece in the soil.

Once you do unearth burdock, you can store it in the refrigerator wrapped in plastic for two weeks. For longer storage, bury it in sand or loamy earth.

Burdock is traditionally harvested in autumn or winter, but you can harvest the thinnings from a spring-sown crop. Soak them in water for twenty minutes and/or parboil to remove any bitterness. Dry them and stir-fry them in sesame cooking oil along with hot peppers sliced in fine threads. Toss with soy sauce and enjoy.

Experiment with burdock. I tried parboiling small roots, then oven-frying as for french fries. Not bad!

Burdock Soup

Combining burdock root with strongly antimicrobial garlic and onion, this soup gives a boost to anyone fighting off infection. Never expecting to like it, I made it for the first time only because of burdock's wonderful healthful properties. Its taste and beautiful caramel color were delightful surprises. Some burdock lovers don't peel burdock root because, they say, the skin has the best flavor. Decide for yourself. In any case, clean the root carefully and cut off any rootlets.

2 teaspoons lemon juice or vinegar

¾ cup burdock root pieces (about an 18-inch piece of root, scrubbed clean and cut into chips as if you were whittling it down, as when sharpening a pencil)

1 leek, sliced into ⅓-inch rounds

1 tablespoon olive oil

¼ cup chopped celery (1 stalk)

1 cup sliced carrots (about 3 carrots)

3 cups chicken broth

4 sprigs of parsley (or 10 stems), chopped

1. Add the lemon juice to 1 quart of water and soak the burdock root pieces for 30 minutes. This will remove bitterness and keep the root from discoloring. Drain the pieces and set aside.

2. Cook the leek rounds in the olive oil until they are limp, about 5 minutes.

3. Add the celery and cook 1 minute; then add the carrots, the burdock root pieces, and the chicken broth.

4. Cook about 25 minutes or until vegetables are soft.

5. Cool slightly, then blend in a blender and return to the pot.

6. Serve hot, garnished with the chopped parsley, or with fried slivers of burdock root or toasted pecans.

YIELD: 8 to 10 servings

TIP

In Japan, burdock root is soaked in vinegar water (2 teaspoons vinegar to 1 quart water) for 30 minutes to remove bitterness and prevent discoloration. Japanese cooks often use the milky water left from washing rice to cook burdock.

Burnet

SANGUISORBA MINOR SYN. POTERIUM SANGUISORBA

BOTANICAL NAME: *Sanguisorba minor,* Rosaceae.

COMMON NAMES: Burnet, salad burnet.

DESCRIPTION: Short-lived perennial.

> *Height:* To 15 inches.
>
> *Flowers:* Green ball flowers with magenta spots.
>
> *Leaves:* Edible, ferny compound leaves on wiry stems.
>
> *Habit:* Low, creeping gradually outward with stems arising from the center.

HARVEST: In spring and fall.

CULTURE: Grow burnet in sunny location in lean, near neutral soil with excellent drainage. It may self-seed in the garden, a good thing because older plants have a tendency to die out.

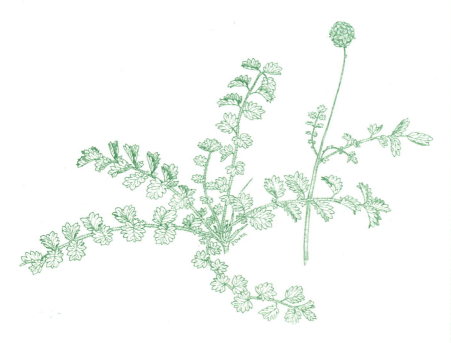

USE: Fresh leaves make a soothing wash for sunburn; leaves have
   styptic properties; great for salads and vinegar.

COMMENTS: A gorgeous, edible garnish. Burnet is very sensitive to
   winter wetness; it makes an outstanding vinegar.

*T*homas Jefferson considered burnet an important "sallet green." Once
you've grown burnet, you'll know why. And you'll wonder why you
didn't grow it sooner.

In the Mid-Atlantic region, where I garden, burnet stays nearly evergreen most years. While I never make a salad from burnet leaves alone, it
is wonderful to have them always available as an interesting addition to
salad or a pretty garnish.

The most delicious cucumber-flavored young leaves are those gathered in spring and fall. The pretty leaves, containing vitamin C, are a
flavorful addition to salads during cool seasons, when they have the fine
cucumber taste. When it gets hot or too cold, the flavor deteriorates.

Burnet, sometimes called "salad burnet" to distinguish it from great
burnet *(Sanguisorba officinalis)*, can be started either in fall or in very early
spring from seed sown a half inch deep. Select a very sunny, well-drained
place where the soil pH is near neutral or even slightly alkaline. Burnet
is hardy in Zones 4 to 9. Lean soil suits it just fine. In fact, if the soil is
too fertile, the plant will grow dense rapidly and need more frequent division. That's fine, too, because the extra plants make a handsome edg-
ing around a salad garden. In early summer, burnet produces unique,
green ball flowers.

If you have a very sunny window, you can also grow salad burnet inside. Inside or out, when the plant begins to look overgrown and di-
sheveled, trim it back for a new, tender supply of leaves. Always harvest
from the center, the source of the youngest, most tender leaves.

Medicinally, salad burnet doesn't have quite the reputation of the
great burnet. However, a fresh leaf may still be used as a styptic to stanch
the flow of blood and as a soothing wash for sunburned skin.

Soothing Burnet Wash

1. Pour 1 cup boiling water over ¼ cup fresh burnet leaves.
2. Allow to steep for 15 minutes.
3. Apply to sunburned skin with cotton balls.

Burnet Vinegar

A classic vinegar, famous for its great flavor. Use leaves picked in fall or spring. If you wash the leaves, make sure they are thoroughly dry.

1 cup burnet leaves on stems (packed)
1 pint bottle white wine vinegar

1. Put burnet leaves in a saucepan and pour the white wine vinegar over them.
2. Heat gently—just to a simmer. Turn off the heat.
3. Let the mixture stand in a covered crock (nonmetal) for a week.
4. Strain the liquid into a bottle that has a cork stopper.

YIELD: 1 pint

TIPS

- *Use burnet as a garnish.*
- *Use burnet in wine cups, potato salad.*
- *Add a few leaves to every salad.*

Caraway

CARUM CARVI

BOTANICAL NAME: *Carum carvi,* Apiaceae.

COMMON NAME: Caraway.

DESCRIPTION: Biennial.

> *Height:* To 2 feet.
>
> *Flowers:* White in loose umbels early in the second summer after planting.
>
> *Leaves:* Fine, carrotlike foliage is edible when young.
>
> *Habit:* Upright, arising from a taproot.

HARVEST: When seeds turn brown.

CULTURE: Easy from seed; may be sown in fall in rich, moist soil that doesn't dry out. Monitor seeds to catch them before they fall.

USE: A safe and gentle digestive used for flatulence, and as a seasoning.

COMMENTS: Edible flowers. Found in prehistoric sites, caraway has been cultivated as a seasoning and medicinal since the Middle Ages.

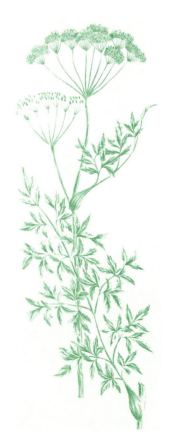

Caraway grows best from fresh seeds that are nigh impossible to come by unless you already have a plant or you have a friend with a plant in seed. To get a start growing this feathery-leaved herb, it's easiest to buy several plants. Set them in a sunny spot in well-drained soil with a nearly neutral pH. You need several, because each plant produces only three or four tablespoons of seeds.

A biennial, in its first year in the garden caraway forms a six-inch mound of carrotlike leaves. It doesn't flower until its second season, when it shoots up two-foot stalks of flat, cream-white flower umbels—not unlike those of Queen Anne's lace. When this happens, begin to monitor your plants. You have to watch for the moment that each tiny flower on the umbel matures into a brown seed capsule. When the capsules on an umbel all turn brown, cut it off. Leave one umbel on the plant to ensure future harvests. When it gets dry enough, its capsules will explode, each shooting two curved caraway seeds into the garden. Keep caraway's long taproot in mind when you reposition the self-sown plants. Transplant carefully and early, while the roots are still small.

Caraway's carrotlike taproot is edible and aromatic snippets of its fine foliage are terrific in salads. Caraway seeds, approved by the German Commission E for dyspeptic complaints, aid digestion and relieve flatulence. Try chewing a half teaspoon of caraway seeds for digestive upset. Or make a tea by pouring a cup of boiling water over a teaspoon of seeds. Allow to steep for ten minutes.

Preparing Caraway Seeds for Culinary Use

The seeds flavor cabbage, cauliflower, potatoes, Irish potato cakes, and baked goods. They can be steeped for a digestive tea. They can also be added to potpourris.

1. Place the freshly harvested caraway seeds in an ovenproof dish or pot.
2. Pour boiling water over the seeds to scald them.
3. Drain the seeds and spread them on a flat tray. Dry them outside in the sun for four days. Bring them in at night.
4. When the seeds are thoroughly dry, store them in an airtight jar.

Caraway Crackers

This recipe is loosely adapted from Estrogen the Natural Way, *by Nina Shandler, who has devised a really neat program for menopausal women who want to replace estrogen without using hormone replacement therapy. I've left in the phytoestrogenic flaxseed, omitted some ingredients, and added others.*

You will have to grind the flaxseed in a coffee grinder.

½ cup flaxseed, ground into flour
¼ cup rye flour
1 tablespoon caraway seeds, divided in half
¾ teaspoon salt, plus additional for sprinkling
½ cup beer (flat is fine) or water
    All-purpose flour as needed (about ½ cup)
    Pepper

1. Preheat the oven to 350°.
2. Combine the flax and rye flours, half the caraway seeds, ¾ teaspoon of the salt, and the beer.
3. Mix together. Add all-purpose flour until the sticky dough can be handled and forms a ball.
4. Allow the dough to rest for 30 minutes. Then knead. Divide into two balls and roll out very thin.
5. Sprinkle the remaining caraway seeds, some salt, and freshly ground pepper over the balls of dough. Use a few strokes of the rolling pin to push these into the dough.
6. Cut the dough into the cracker sizes you wish.
7. Line a cookie sheet with parchment paper, reduce heat to 325°, and bake for 20 to 25 minutes, or until dry and crackerlike.

YIELD: 40 crackers (1.5″ diameter)

The Thyme Garden's Harissa

In addition to an array of culinary and medicinal herbs, the Thyme Garden Herb Seed Company includes some excellent recipes in its catalog (see Sources). This one combines seeds—caraway, cumin, and coriander—with mint and chilis for a spicy Middle Eastern sauce or marinade that's great with any barbecued or grilled meat. Use a coffee grinder to grind the seeds. The difference between preground and freshly ground is amazing.

2 ounces dried red chilis (or less—the amount of heat is up to you)
2 cloves garlic
1 teaspoon crumbled dried mint
1 teaspoon freshly ground caraway seeds
2 teaspoons freshly ground cumin seeds
2 teaspoons freshly ground coriander seeds
2 tablespoons extra-virgin olive oil

1. Seed the chilis, tear them into pieces, and soak them in warm water until they are soft—about 20 minutes.
2. While the chilis are soaking, peel, crush, and pound the garlic with a mortar and pestle, or process the peeled cloves in a food processor.
3. Pound or process the chilis and the mint with the garlic.
4. Mix in the ground seeds. Add the olive oil to form a paste.

When ready to use, coat the meat and let it marinate for at least 3 hours.

YIELD: Enough for 1 to 1½ pounds of meat

TIP

Add caraway seeds to cabbage water to reduce odor.

Carrot

DAUCUS CAROTA

BOTANICAL NAME: *Daucus carota,* Apiaceae.

COMMON NAME: Carrot.

DESCRIPTION: Root vegetable grown as an annual.

Height: To 12 inches.

Flowers: If unharvested, Queen Anne's lace–type flowers in second year.

Leaves: Finely cut, bright green, arise from the underground carrot.

HARVEST: Dig carrots before the ground freezes. Cut the tops back to just under an inch. They can be left outside, stacked between layers of leaves or peat moss under an upturned box, or stored in a cold basement or garage (between 32 and 40 degrees Fahrenheit), or, if you have room, in the refrigerator.

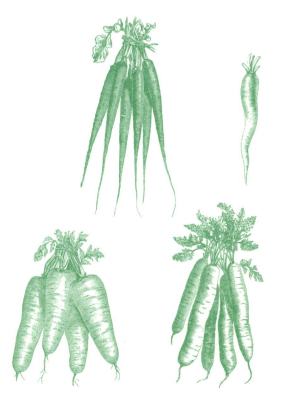

CULTURE: In Zones 4 to 7, start in early spring; in Zones 8 and 9, grow over winter. Rich, loose soil in full sun to very light shade.

Companionable plants, carrots are good companions to grow with lettuce, onions, marigolds, parsley, and thyme.

USE: Carrots contain the antioxidants alpha- and beta-carotene and are a highly nutritious vegetable.

COMMENTS: Eat carrots every day. Some research suggests that while eating raw carrots is good for you, cooked, juiced, or puréed is even better.

*E*verything Grandma said they were, carrots have it all—antioxidants, fiber, and eight compounds that lower blood pressure. Beta-carotene in carrots enhances the action of natural killer cells called lymphocytes that can destroy tumors. If you want to reduce your chances of stroke, cancer, and high blood pressure and preserve your eyesight, liver, and general well-being, grow your own carrots. Because carrots can absorb heavy metal residues and traces of pesticides from soil that contains these toxins, grow them organically to make sure that these root vegetables are free of toxins. Then eat some every day.

According to the Seeds of Change catalog (see Sources), the heirloom carrot "St. Valery" has the "highest amount of free arginine" (a protein-building amino acid) among those tested. Still another carrot, "Marche de Paris," is harvestable when very small, and thus is suitable for container gardening.

If you don't object to planting hybrids, you may wish to try one of the new supercarrots. Seed catalogs offer a wonderful variety. For sheer taste, try "Sweetness II," as sweet as its name. "BetaSweet" is not only sweeter than average, but contains ample beta-carotene. "Artist" is a carrot with higher-than-average vitamin A content. There are no bad carrots.

Not everybody has the right sort of soil in which to grow carrots. I didn't at first. I had clay soil and failed miserably until I amended one part of my garden specifically for carrot culture. Digging the soil to a depth of eighteen inches, I added the finest grade of chicken grit, sand, and as much compost and organic material as I could get my hands on.

Carrots with Rosemary Butter

Hot grated carrots with rosemary butter are an extremely simple and delicious way to load up on antioxidants. Don't sweat the butter. According to John Erdman, director of nutritional sciences at the University of Illinois in Urbana, beta-carotene needs a small amount of fat to get through the intestinal wall into the body.

FOR THE ROSEMARY BUTTER:
¼ pound unsalted butter, softened
2 tablespoons finely chopped rosemary

FOR THE CARROTS:
6 carrots, grated and very lightly salted
2 tablespoons rosemary butter (see step 1)
Salt
Pepper

1. Combine the butter and rosemary to make ¼ pound of rosemary butter. Set aside.
2. Microwave the carrots in a covered dish for approximately 3 minutes, or until softened and bright orange.
3. Toss the carrots with 2 tablespoons of the rosemary butter. Add salt and pepper to taste.

YIELD: 4 servings

A. Brockie Stevenson's
Dilled, Chilled Carrot Soup

Everyone loves this soup—even people who don't usually eat carrots. Artist Brockie Stevenson gave me the recipe for this delicious and beautiful soup, and it is forever entwined in my mind with summer and the hard-edged, clean lines of the clapboard houses that inhabit his paintings and silkscreen prints. As cooling as the breeze off Penobscot Bay, the soup is a splendid make-ahead first course for a sum-mer dinner party. I often keep a pitcher of it in the refrigerator for a low-calorie combination of antiaging, antioxidant carrots and soothing, easy-to-digest dill.

    1 leek, chopped (about 2 cups), or 2 onions, cut into sixths
    1 tablespoon olive oil
  6–8 large carrots, cut into 1-inch chunks (about 3 cups)
    2 stalks of celery, roughly chopped (about ¾ cup)
    4 cups (or 2 cans) chicken broth
    2 tablespoons fresh dill plus some for garnish
    1 teaspoon salt, or to taste
      Freshly ground black pepper

1. Cook the leek in the olive oil until it is soft.
2. Add the carrots, celery, chicken broth, 2 tablespoons of the dill, and salt.
3. Cook all the ingredients together until the vegetables are soft, about 20 minutes.
4. Cool slightly. Purée in batches in a blender.
5. Taste and adjust the seasoning.
6. Chill for at least 3 hours. (May also be served hot.)
7. Pour into bowls. Garnish with the remaining dill. Sprinkle liberally with the pepper.

YIELD: 4 to 6 servings

Chamomile

MATRICARIA RECUTITA; CHAMAEMELUM NOBILE

BOTANICAL NAME: *Matricaria recutita,* Asteraceae.

COMMON NAMES: Chamomile, German chamomile.

DESCRIPTION: An annual that reseeds.

> *Height:* To 18 inches.
>
> *Flowers:* Small, white, daisy-like flowers in late spring, summer.
>
> *Leaves:* Ferny.

HARVEST: Gather the flowers, when they are open, in dry, sunny weather; dry them on screens in an airy place.

CULTURE: Grow chamomile in full sun and well-drained soil.

USE: A tea from the flowers is soothing to the nerves and digestive system.

COMMENTS: Chamomile self-sows. Hay fever sufferers should avoid this herb. Chamomile belongs to the same family as ragweed and may cause allergic reactions in susceptible individuals. Pregnant women should avoid this herb just to be on the safe side.

BOTANICAL NAME: *Chamaemelum nobile,* Asteraceae.

COMMON NAME: Roman chamomile.

DESCRIPTION: Perennial herb.

> *Height:* To 6 inches.
>
> *Flowers:* Small, daisy-like flowers.
>
> *Leaves:* Very fine, bright green.

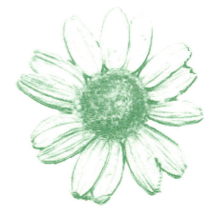

HARVEST: Gather flowers as soon as they open.

CULTURE: Grow Roman chamomile in full sun in light, well-drained soil.

USE: Chamomile flowers make a tea that is helpful for digestive disorders. Externally, chamomile extract is soothing to irritated skin.

COMMENTS: Roman chamomile dies back in areas that are hot in summer. Hay fever sufferers should approach chamomile, a relative of ragweed, with caution.

*T*wo very similar plants, used interchangeably, are called chamomile. One, Roman chamomile *(Chamaemelum nobile),* is a perennial that thrives where summers are cool—alas, not where I live. This is the one famed for use as a lawn. If you live in a climate with cool summers, you can plant perennial Roman chamomile once and enjoy it for a good long time. Where summers are hot, it may die back over the summer, to return when the weather cools off.

Roman chamomile forms mats of short, fine, apple-scented foliage. A nonflowering cultivar called "Treneague" is great for use as a lawn. It's no good medicinally, however, because the effective part of the plant is the flower.

German chamomile *(Matricaria recutita)* is an annual that thrives in heat. Unscathed by hot, humid summers, it self-sows all over. This is a good thing, because you need at least six large plants to have enough flowers to dry for a winter's worth of tea. A well-grown plant produces at least fifteen flowers per day—about half the amount needed for one cup of tea.

Somehow chamomile volunteers are never a nuisance. Not only do they produce more flowers for a soothing tea, they dress up the garden. Pretty tufts of bright green, ferny leaves, studded with golden-centered, small, white daisy-like flowers, always seem to pop up in places that need adornment. The sites these volunteers select for themselves—often hot spots where little else survives—support specimens that grow larger and produce more flowers. Chamomile is altogether welcome in my garden, wherever it appears.

Start seeds of annual German chamomile in fall or very early spring by scattering them on the ground in a sunny place with light, dryish soil. They grow quickly, and if your growing season is long, you will have more than one generation.

Well-known as a sedative tea made from the flowers, chamomile also contains powerful anti-inflammatory compounds and can be used topically. Its medicinal history is long and impressive. In ancient Egypt it was given for malarial fevers. Dioscorides and Pliny valued it. It figures in Ayurvedic medicine. In nineteenth-century America, it was recommended for just about every ailment.

Recent research supports tradition: chamomile contains compounds that depress the central nervous system and relax smooth muscle. One study has shown it to be as effectual as an opium-based drug without the side effects. For this reason, a tea from its flowers is a gentle nightcap that conveys antianxiety and antistress properties. It also aids digestion. A variety that contains very high levels of the active pharmacological components is *Matricaria recutita* 'Bona,' also very early to flower.

Although chamomile is on the FDA's list of plants that are generally safe, because it is a member of the same family that includes ragweed, anyone who suffers from hay fever should avoid this plant or approach it with extreme caution. It is not recommended for pregnant women.

Harvesting Chamomile Flowers for Tea

1. Chamomile flowers arrive in a great burst in late spring, and then appear intermittently all summer. This means you harvest all summer long. The more you harvest, the more flowers will be produced, because none will have gone to seed.
2. Take a daily walk through the garden after the dew has dried. Pick off just the heads of freshly opened flowers. Each time you gather about sixteen of them, you've earned yourself another cup of pure chamomile tea or the makings of a blend.
3. Place these out of the sun in a warm, airy place to dry. I use an upturned basket in the dining room, close to the garden door.

4. Check the drying flowers regularly. I find that the dense centers hold moisture far longer than one would expect. Before storing, if there's any doubt whatsoever, pour the flowers onto a tray and dry them in an oven that has been warmed, but turned off, until they are thoroughly dry. Store the dried flowers in a jar.

Sleep Tea

1 cup dried chamomile flowers
½ cup dried lemon balm leaves
1 dropperful Knockout Decoction (page 253)

1. Mix the flowers and leaves well and store in an airtight jar, out of the light.
2. For tea, put 2 teaspoons of the mix into a teapot.
3. Add 10 ounces boiling water.
4. Steep for 7 minutes.
5. Add the Knockout Decoction and sleep well.

Chamomile Under-Eye Oil

After buying a similar oil that came in a teeny bottle with an enormous price tag, I experimented with making my own. This simple recipe works well. I use it to gently bleach the skin under my eyes and smooth wrinkles. For the oil, I chose jojoba, but almond or olive oil would work, too.

½ cup packed dried chamomile flowers
4 ounces good-quality oil suitable for use on the skin
1 tablespoon lemon juice

1. Pack the flowers into a jar large enough to hold them with a bit of headroom.
2. Completely cover the flowers with the oil. Add a half inch or so over

the top to make sure flowers don't stick out (at first they may float, but when they become thoroughly moistened, they sink).

3. Place the jar in a sunny window for a week. Strain. Add the lemon juice. Mix thoroughly and put a small amount in a tiny bottle for immediate use. Refrigerate the rest. Use within a month.

Chaste Tree

VITEX AGNUS-CASTUS

BOTANICAL NAME: *Vitex agnus-castus,* Verbenaceae.

COMMON NAME: Chaste tree.

DESCRIPTION: A deciduous shrub or small tree.

> *Height:* To 20 feet.
>
> *Flowers:* Purple in terminal spikes in summer; 'Alba,' a white form, and 'Rosea,' a pink form, are available.
>
> *Leaves:* Neatly cut, gray-green, bird's-foot-shaped leaves.
>
> *Habit:* Rather stiff, branching into a rounded shape.

HARVEST: Berries when hard and dry.

CULTURE: Zone 6 to 8 (and worth a try in Zone 5). Site in sun, in ordinary soil with good drainage.

USE: Berries are used in tinctures and teas to normalize hormone function.

COMMENTS: A handsome addition to the home landscape where hardy; at the limits of its hardiness, stems may die back to the roots, but because it blooms on the current year's wood, this is not critical. In fact, chaste tree makes a handsome cut-back shrub.

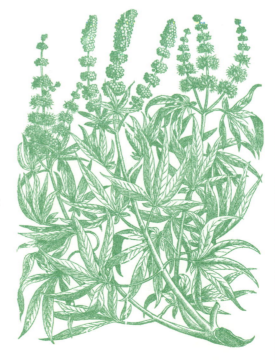

CAUTION: Overdosing (much more than the recommended dose of 1 to 3 dropperfuls of liquid extract per day) causes a condition called formication—the sensation of ants crawling over the skin.

*C*haste tree grows to about twenty feet high in California and the South, but at the northern edges of its hardiness range (it is rated Zone 6) it is really an ornamental shrub. Everything about this plant is appealing. Its aromatic, bird's-foot leaves are held on rather stiff branches that give the shrub pleasing volume. Late-summer flowers, at the tips of the branches, are pale lilac and fragrant.

Of Mediterranean origin, it is easy to grow in soil of ordinary fertility as long as it has a sunny position. In dry climates, it thrives with extra watering as long as it has good drainage. Chaste tree needs sun and heat to produce flowers and berries.

The medicinal parts of this plant are the dusty blue-black berries. From them comes the name chaste tree, which refers to their reputation as inhibitors of sexual passion. Their former use in monasteries to suppress libido earned chaste tree another common name, "monk's pepper."

Today, herbalists value chaste tree as a women's herb to restore hormonal balance. Numerous studies support chaste tree's efficacy in regulating menstruation, diminishing mastalgia (breast tenderness), and treating the symptoms of PMS and menopause. It is on the approved list of the German Commission E for treating menstrual irregularities.

The best results are from long-term use of chaste tree. The results are not so much dramatic changes as they are simply a return to normal. For example, if a patient suffers from lack of menses or from abnormally heavy bleeding, chaste tree works by restoring regularity or diminishing the flow.

One of the country's most highly respected herbalists, Christopher Hobbs, recommends vitex for acne in teenagers. As with many herbal remedies, the effects are not instantaneous, but require a month or two of treatment before results are seen.

Hormone-Balance Tincture

Making a tincture sounded like something terribly esoteric that I would never do. But it couldn't have been easier. Now I stock food-grade alcohol, purchased from a liquor store (brands include Clear Spring and Everclear), so that I can whip one up when the right ingredients are available. Vodka is an alternative to food-grade alcohol. Never use rubbing alcohol. Often, small brown bottles with dropper tops are available where bulk herbs are sold (see Sources). Tinctures retain their effectiveness for a year or more.

    1 ounce (28 grams) dried vitex berries
  280 milliliters 190-proof food-grade alcohol (available in liquor stores)

1. Grind the vitex berries in a coffee grinder.
2. Place the powder in the bottom of a jelly jar.
3. Pour the alcohol over the ground berries. Put the lid on the jar and shake thoroughly.
4. Shake once or twice a day for a month.
5. Strain the mixture through a coffee filter. Pour into bottles. Store out of the light.

NOTE: Take 35 drops—about a dropperful—or ¼ teaspoon of the tincture daily in juice to disguise the flavor. Don't take more or it will make your skin feel unpleasantly prickly.

Chervil

ANTHRISCUS CEREFOLIUM

BOTANICAL NAME: *Anthriscus cerefolium,* Apiaceae.

COMMON NAMES: Chervil, French parsley.

DESCRIPTION: Annual.

> *Height:* To 2 feet.
>
> *Flowers:* Umbels of small white flowers.
>
> *Leaves:* Light green, parsleylike leaves with a mildly anise flavor.

HARVEST: Cut chervil as needed; cut mature plants and preserve as pesto.

CULTURE: Chervil requires cool, moist soil in sun to part shade with cool air temperatures; as a pot plant it thrives at around 60 degrees Fahrenheit in a sunny window.

USE: A tea made with chervil leaves can be used in a gentle compress for the eyes; chervil is an ingredient in fines herbes.

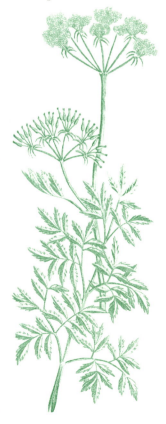

COMMENTS: Edible flowers. Cut off flowers as they form to encourage the production of new leaves.

I think of chervil as happy-go-lucky parsley's delicate, high-strung cousin. It is an annual herb that grows lushly only when conditions are perfect—rich, moist, well-drained soil in a cool place in morning sun or partial shade.

There's a window of cool weather on either end of summer and that's the time to grow chervil, unless you are lucky enough to have a cold frame to keep it going over winter. Barring that, a window that gets plenty of sun in a room that stays cool—ideally 60 degrees Fahrenheit—will keep chervil happy in a container.

Chervil comes up quickly from seed (but resents transplanting) and will flower in eight weeks. Harvest leaves from the outside of the plant when it is at least four weeks old and before it blooms. Pinch off any flower buds to promote more foliage.

Chervil has been used as a treatment for conjunctivitis and as an ingredient in spring tonics. By far its most cherished attribute is an anise flavor that is so delicate it must be added at the end of cooking. Sprinkle fresh, chopped leaves over hot carrots, tomatoes, or peas. Sometimes included in mesclun mixes, chervil is also an essential ingredient in fines herbes.

Fines Herbes Oil

Freezing a mixture of fresh fines herbes blended in oil is a great way to preserve the herbs' flavor. Dry the herbs carefully before blending in olive oil.

½ cup chervil sprigs, washed and completely dry
½ cup whole chives, washed and completely dry
½ cup tarragon leaves, washed and completely dry
1 cup Italian parsley sprigs, washed and completely dry
½ cup olive oil, or enough to keep the mixture from sticking in the blender

1. Blend all the ingredients.
2. Refrigerate the amount intended for immediate use.
3. Freeze some for later.

> **TIP**
>
> *Do not dry chervil leaves, as they lose their flavor and fade. Blend instead with a little olive oil for a thick pesto and freeze.*

Chives

ALLIUM SCHOENOPRASUM

BOTANICAL NAME: *Allium schoenoprasum,* Liliaceae.

COMMON NAME: Chive.

DESCRIPTION: A perennial onion, grown for the leaf.

> *Height:* To 1 foot.

> *Flowers:* The pink pom-pom flowers are edible.

> *Leaves:* Narrow, hollow, tubular leaves with a fine onion flavor.

HARVEST: Cut close to the ground as needed; preserve in olive oil and vinegar.

CULTURE: Zones 3 to 10. Plant in moist, well-drained, neutral, fertile soil. Makes a good windowsill plant. Divide every three years and replant into soil enriched with compost. Chives deter aphids and make good companions to carrots, lettuce, roses, and tomatoes.

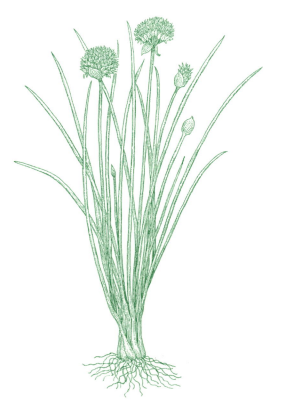

USE: Chives are a gentle supplier of some of the same sulfur compounds as onions and are invaluable in the kitchen.

COMMENTS: Rather than trying to neaten the plant after it flowers, cut it back to the ground to ensure a continual supply of the flavorful leaves. It will come back—fast!

*U*nlike most of their onion cousins, chives are grown for their green leaves, not their bulbous roots. Even so, chives share some of the nutritional and medicinal virtues of the onion family: vitamins and iron, and sulfur compounds.

Chives are easy to grow on a windowsill, where they will be readily available. Snip the hollow stems at the soil level and add to soups, salads, or vegetables. For best results, pot chives up before the first frost and allow the plants a month or so of dormancy before bringing them in.

Inside, give them sun or strong light and moist well-drained soil. Outside, they seem to thrive anywhere, even in dampish, partly shaded places. Growing about a foot tall, they spread into large colonies that are studded with pink pom-pom flowers that make a pretty, edible garnish—either fresh or dried—for salads and soups. The flower stalks, hard as pencils, are inedible. The flexible leaves make charming presentations on the plate when they are used to tie bundles of green beans or carrot strips.

Chive Vinaigrette

Make this vinaigrette in the blender for a foamy texture and fine chartreuse color. It's an easy dressed-up vinaigrette for a special presentation. Try it as a color-coordinated and tasty dressing with cold artichoke hearts.

- ¾ cup olive oil
- 2 tablespoons white wine vinegar
- 2 tablespoons chopped chives (about ten 12-inch blades)
- 1 tablespoon chopped Italian parsley
- 2–4 lemon balm leaves

> **TIP**
>
> *P*ick the chive flowers to use their peppery-onion flavor. Separate the pink pom-poms into small bits and toss them in a salad or mix with cream cheese.

½ teaspoon chopped shallots
¼ teaspoon dry mustard
   Salt and pepper

1. Combine all the ingredients in a blender.
2. Blend to a foamy yellow-green.

YIELD: 1 cup

Salmon "Scallopini" with Chive Cream

One of the delights of my life is to take a class at l'Academie de Cuisine in suburban Washington, D.C., and watch chef François Dionot at work. Over the years, I have incorporated his tenets into my cooking. His is the voice in my head that guides me as I cook—scolding me if I attempt a shortcut, advising to season as I go, to always use sea salt and unsalted butter. This, like all of his recipes, is richly delicious.

1 pound salmon fillets
   Peanut oil or extra-virgin olive oil
   Fresh chives (about ¾ cup)
½ cup crème fraîche or sour cream
   Salt and pepper
   Juice of 1 lemon

1. Slice the salmon fillets into thin pieces, 2–3 per person. Place the slices on a lightly oiled baking sheet.
2. Reserving some for garnish, finely chop the chives and mix into the crème fraîche. Add salt, pepper, and lemon juice to taste.
3. Brush the salmon with the crème fraîche mixture, enough to cover the fish well. Set aside, or refrigerate if preparing ahead of time.
4. Preheat the broiler. Minutes before serving, place the salmon under a hot broiler for 1 to 1½ minutes.
5. Decorate with a colorful garnish of chives.

YIELD: 4 servings

Cilantro, Coriander

CORIANDRUM SATIVUM

BOTANICAL NAME: *Coriandrum sativum,* Apiaceae.

COMMON NAMES: Cilantro, coriander.

DESCRIPTION: Annual.

Height: To 12+ feet.

Flowers: White or pink in hot weather; these are followed by the round, light brown seeds.

Leaves: Deep green, parsley-shaped leaves with a distinctive aroma.

HARVEST: Leaves at any time; seeds when they turn tan.

CULTURE: Cool, moist soil keeps the leaves coming; hot conditions bring the plant into flower and, ultimately, seed. Siting near fennel is said to inhibit cilantro's growth.

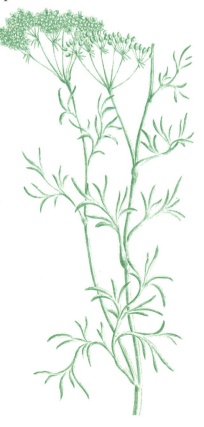

USE: Leaves and seeds make a tea that aids in digestion and alleviates flatulence; appetite stimulant; antiallergen; eye wash.

COMMENTS: 'Slo-Bolt' is a variety that is slow to come into flower and that thus lasts longer in the garden.

"Cilantro" is the Spanish name for coriander and has come to refer to the green leaves of this plant, while "coriander" refers more frequently to the seeds. A distinctive and essential ingredient in Mexican, Southwestern, and Asian cuisine, cilantro produces leaves, seeds, and roots that flavor curries and many other dishes. It yields a tea that aids in digestion and alleviates flatulence.

Cilantro has leaves shaped like those of Italian parsley, but its flavor is like nothing else. People either love it or hate it. If you are among the former, you have plenty of company. Coriander seeds have been found in ancient pharaonic tombs. The Greeks and Romans used the plant medicinally, and in Ayurvedic medicine cilantro is used in eyewashes and is indicated for a host of ailments, including allergies and urinary problems. In traditional Chinese medicine it is an aphrodisiac. The German Commission E approved coriander seed as an appetite stimulant and for dyspepsia.

Sown in moist, well-drained soil in a sunny place, cilantro, an annual, comes up easily from seed. Maintaining a steady supply of the pungent leaves is more challenging, because plants from a spring sowing go to seed as soon as the weather turns hot. To keep leaves coming, you can keep replanting seed, but it's far easier to wait for cool weather.

I have found that cilantro does better even on a windowsill over the winter than it does in the summer garden. The place where cilantro absolutely luxuriates over winter is in a cold frame. If you have one and you love this herb, a cold frame is the perfect place to start the cilantro cycle rolling. Spring-sown plants go to seed in midsummer, germinate in fall, and provide plenty of greens all winter long. Just before flowering and going to seed, cilantro grows tall, with fine, feathery leaves. Collect the seed and use a coffee grinder to make your own coriander powder. Cilantro is an essential in my kitchen.

Curry in a Hurry

I could never understand how my friend Rabia Hussein, a busy scientist, was able to throw dinner parties so frequently and so well. I can remember the tantalizing aromas of her dishes wafting out into the hall as I knocked at her door. Be-

fore she returned to Pakistan, she taught me her secret. She would make and freeze the following mixture to give a base flavor to many of her dishes. I use it for everything—as seasoning for a marinade, as a base for curries, and in soups. It is outstanding as a flavoring for lentils.

    2 medium onions, cut into chunks
 6–8 cloves garlic, peeled
       5-inch piece of ginger, peeled and chunked
 1–2 (depending upon how hot you like your curry) green chilis,
       seeds removed
    1 bunch cilantro (about a cup)
       Water to facilitate blending, about ½ cup

1. Blend all the ingredients together in a blender.
2. Add just enough water to keep the blender moving.

NOTE: You will have close to two cups of Curry in a Hurry. You can use 2 tablespoons for Curried Lentils (recipe follows). Freeze the rest in ¼-cup portions in freezer bags or in recycled yogurt containers.

Curried Lentils

Even if you don't ordinarily like lentils, try this dish. It may change your mind.

    2 cups (1 pound) red lentils
    2 tablespoons olive oil
    2 tablespoons Curry in a Hurry (see recipe above)
    2 teaspoons curry powder
    2 cups (or 1 can) chicken broth
    ½ teaspoon salt plus additional to taste
    4 ounces coconut milk, mixed well
       Up to ½ cup water

1. Pick over and wash the lentils. Put them in a pot with a quart of water and bring to a boil. Turn down the heat and simmer 5 minutes. Remove from heat.

2. Heat the olive oil in the bottom of a large pot. Add the Curry in a Hurry. Cook for 3 minutes. Add the curry powder. Cook for 1 minute.

3. Add the drained lentils, the chicken broth, and ½ teaspoon of the salt. Cover and simmer slowly for 10 minutes.

4. Add the coconut milk. Stir and cook another 2 or 3 minutes. If the soup is too thick, add ½ cup water or chicken stock if you have it. Salt to taste.

YIELD: 6 to 8 servings

Black Bean–Cornmeal Muffins with Cilantro

Cilantro is one of the spices that give these savory muffins a south-of-the-border flavor. In working out this recipe, I discovered that the crucial step was omitting the sugar that is usually asked for in corn bread recipes. The taste should be savory—a welcome change from sweet rolls for breakfast. Black bean–cornmeal muffins can be as spicy as you like, depending upon the type of pepper added. Great with huevos rancheros, these muffins are also good as a take-to-the-office snack with guacamole or cut in half for a tomato-avocado sandwich. Nutritious in its own right, cornmeal marries happily with beans, onions, peppers, cilantro, and tomatoes for muffins that abound in phytochemicals to protect against breast and colon cancers.

1¼ cups all-purpose flour

¾ cup cornmeal

2 teaspoons baking powder

1¾ teaspoons sea salt

1 cup skim milk

¼ cup vegetable oil

1 egg, beaten

¾ teaspoon ground cumin

¾ teaspoon dried oregano

2 tablespoons finely chopped onion

1–2 medium tomatoes, chopped and drained
2 tablespoons finely chopped fresh cilantro
1 teaspoon finely chopped hot green chili
⅔ cup cooked black beans, drained
2 ounces (½ cup) shredded Monterey Jack

1. Preheat oven to 400°. Grease and flour a muffin tin.
2. In a large bowl, mix together the flour, cornmeal, baking powder, sea salt, milk, vegetable oil, egg, cumin, and oregano.
3. Fold in the onion, tomatoes, cilantro, and chili, and, gently, the beans and cheese.
4. Pour this batter into the muffin tin.
5. Bake 20 to 25 minutes, or until the muffins are a light golden brown and a fork inserted in the center comes out clean.

YIELD: 12 muffins

> ### TIP
>
> * *To keep cilantro fresh, place the stems in water.*
> * *Don't throw away cilantro roots; they can be used for flavoring curries and stews.*

Dandelion

TARAXACUM OFFICINALE

BOTANICAL NAME: *Taraxacum officinale,* Asteraceae.

COMMON NAME: Dandelion.

DESCRIPTION: Perennial.

>*Height:* To 1 foot.

>*Flowers:* Yellow; may be made into wine.

>*Leaves:* Notched; medium green in a low rosette.

HARVEST: Leaves are least bitter in early spring; gather roots in fall as a vegetable or for roasting.

CULTURE: Zones 3 to 10. Easy; average soil; sun to part shade.

USE: Diuretic, blood purifier, nutritionally superior green.

COMMENTS: Never eat dandelions from a lawn treated with pesticides.

OTHER SPECIES: Italian dandelion, or chicory *(Cichorium intybus),* with similar properties.

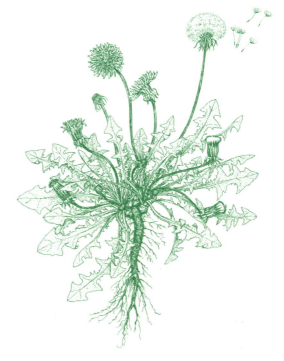

$\mathcal{M}$ost homeowners do their best to kill dandelions. Yet the same plants that people try to eradicate from lawns are not merely edible, they are nutritionally incredible. Unless you treat your lawn with pesticides or so-called lawn food that contains preemergent weed killer, chances are you are already growing a crop of dandelions. All you have to do is pick the leaves. The best time to do this is in the spring before they become bitter. *Never* eat dandelions from a lawn that has been treated with pesticides.

Dandelion's botanical name *Taraxacum* means "remedy for disorders," and this plant is on the German Commission E's approved list for dyspeptic conditions. Medicinally, dandelions are used as a diuretic, as an aid to digestion (to reduce bloating), and as an effective blood purifier to assist in healing eczema and acne. Dandelions may even help to prevent breast cancer. In order to benefit from them, you don't have to make a tincture or tea; all you have to do is eat the leaves, cooked or in salads, or the young roots, cooked like parsnips.

Nutrient powerhouses, ounce for ounce dandelions contain more vitamin A than broccoli, chard, collards, spinach, or carrots—to say nothing of some of their other components, which include vitamin B complex, vitamins C and E, calcium, magnesium, potash, and zinc. One would think that with their hefty load of vitamins and minerals and their medicinal properties, they would be more highly prized in this country. The problem is their bitter taste.

Mixing dandelion greens with other ingredients cancels out the bitterness. Try them mixed with other greens, or in lasagna (recipes follow).

Dandelions are far more popular in French gardens, and the French have developed strains for culinary use. One of these, 'Pissenlit Improved,' uses the French common name for dandelion. Roughly translated, *pissenlit* means "wet the bed" and refers to the use of dandelion root as a diuretic.

Any plant as ubiquitous as the dandelion is likely to be easy to grow, but there are a few things to keep in mind. Dandelions are one of those plants that cause the premature maturation of other plants by exhaling ethylene gas—consider giving one part of your plot over to dandelion culture. You can start seeds early in spring for spring and summer greens or in early summer for fall and winter eating. Sow seeds thinly, because most will come up. Even though the package will say it takes about ninety days for the plants to mature, you can harvest the leaves as soon as you think it is worth it. And the thinnings are good in salads and soups, or cooked separately. Boil the roots until they are tender and season them with salt and pepper.

Dandelion greens are bitter to begin with and become more bitter as the growing season advances. One way to keep the leaves sweet is to blanch them by tying the outside leaves together early in the plant's life and allowing them to develop out of full sunlight. Otherwise, to sweeten picked greens, boil briefly, discard the water, and then cook them as you would spinach.

Italian dandelion, or chicory *(Cichorium intybus)*, is a perennial, growing to maturity in forty-eight days from seed. As with dandelions, its bitter taste mixes well with potatoes and onions.

Dandelion Root Tea

1. Bring 1¼ cups water to a boil.
2. Add 2 teaspoons dried dandelion root. Turn the heat down and cover.
3. Allow to simmer for 15 minutes.
4. Strain and drink.

Dandelion Lasagna with Shiitakes

If you don't spray your lawn, you've already got some of the ingredients for this lasagna variation. I've been making lasagna with spinach for years. It was a short jump to dandelions—there for the picking. For this recipe, I use a 6 × 10-inch pan to make enough for four moderately hungry people. Adjust this forgiving recipe to suit your cookware.

    6 lasagna noodles (for 3 layers)
  5–6 shiitake mushroom caps, chopped
    ½ tablespoon butter
    1 large onion, chopped fine
    1 tablespoon olive oil
  3–4 cups of dandelion leaves, washed and picked clean of grass

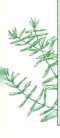

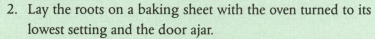

HOW TO ROAST DANDELION ROOTS

1. Cut off the leaves and scrub the roots.
2. Lay the roots on a baking sheet with the oven turned to its lowest setting and the door ajar.
3. It may take 3 to 4 hours until the roots are shriveled and snap easily. They are done when the insides of the roots are dark brown.

Salt and pepper
1 carton (16-ounce) cottage cheese or ricotta, nonfat if you like
2 eggs, beaten
¼ cup chopped parsley
1 can/jar (26-ounce) spaghetti sauce
2 ounces Gruyère, grated

1. Cook the lasagna noodles, drain them, and set them aside in cold water until ready to use.
2. Sauté the shiitakes in the butter and set them aside.
3. Cook the chopped onion in olive oil until it is softened. Add the dandelion leaves. Season with salt and pepper. Cook until dark green and limp, about 5 minutes.
4. Preheat the oven to 350°.
5. Mix the cottage cheese with the 2 beaten eggs. Add the chopped parsley. Season with salt and pepper.
6. Spoon a ¼-inch layer of the spaghetti sauce into the bottom of the pan. Lay 2 lasagna noodles over it side by side. Add a hefty layer of sauce. Lay 2 noodles on top of the sauce.
7. Add all of the cottage cheese mixture as the next layer. Arrange the dandelions and onions evenly over the top. Cover with the remaining 2 noodles.
8. Add more spaghetti sauce. Top with the shiitakes and Gruyère.
9. Bake for about 30 minutes.

YIELD: 4 servings

Jan Midgley's Classic Greens

Jan Midgley is a gardening chum who grew up in Missouri eating Southern-style, down-home cooking. This classic recipe has a down-home flavor that's hard to beat—and hard to get without adding plenty of bacon fat. This recipe uses none. It is presented here complete with Jan's asides and in the vernacular.

1 grocery plastic sack of mixed greens (collard [see note], kale, turnip, rape, mustard, and dandelion greens)
1 tablespoon olive oil
1 small onion, chopped
1 clove garlic, chopped or mashed (as in "mash that button")
¼ cup chicken stock or water
½ cube Knorr ham bouillon
Sugar, a generous pinch
Salt and black pepper
1 teaspoon hot pepper vinegar, or to taste

NOTE: Need to steam for 4 minutes longer than the other greens.

1. Rinse the greens and place them in a colander (do not spin dry). Remove tough stems (leave some of the stem for texture if it isn't too tough).
2. Stack 8 to 10 leaves like a deck of cards on a cutting board. Fold in half along the rib and cut into strips about 1 inch wide.
3. Place the prepared greens in a large bowl, keeping the collards separate from the others.
4. Heat a large skillet (one with a lid) to medium or medium high and put the olive oil into it.
5. Sauté the onion and garlic just until the onion is clear. If the garlic starts to get more than golden brown, don't worry about whether the onion is cooked. It will finish cooking while the greens cook.
6. Immediately pile in the greens: if using collards, add them first and cook for 4 minutes, covered. Then add the rest of the greens and sauté and turn for 5 minutes.

7. If there isn't enough liquid on the greens to produce some steam with the lid on, add the stock or water now. Cook, covered, on low heat for 7 to 10 minutes.

8. Add the chicken stock (if you haven't already done so), bouillon cube, sugar (it removes any bitterness, as it does for boiled turnip root), and salt and pepper. Stir well. Just before removing from the heat, sprinkle the hot pepper vinegar over the dish and turn the greens to distribute the flavoring.

YIELD: 4 servings

Dill

ANETHUM GRAVEOLENS

BOTANICAL NAME: *Anethum graveolens,* Apiaceae.

COMMON NAMES: Dill, dill weed.

DESCRIPTION: Annual.

> *Height:* To 6 feet.
>
> *Flowers:* Yellow umbels in summer; edible seeds follow.
>
> *Leaves:* Aromatic, soft, ferny.

HARVEST: Greens at any time. Cut seed heads and allow them to finish ripening in paper bags. Leaves lose flavor quickly when dry. Freeze or store in salt (see Mrs. Adams's Salt Method for Preserving Dill, page 69).

CULTURE: Sow seed where it is to grow in moist, fertile, slightly acid soil; do successive sowings to keep greens coming. Dill is a good companion to cabbage, lettuce, and onions.

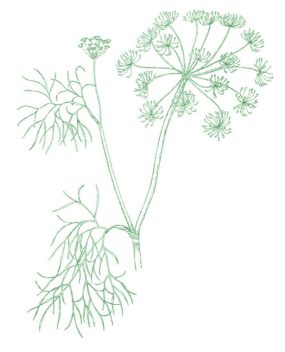

USE: Seeds are a digestive, used in combating flatulence; they inhibit growth of *E. coli* bacteria. Seeds and greens are a seasoning.

COMMENTS: Site tall dill north of shorter herbs.

The word "dill" comes from an Old Norse word meaning "to soothe." And that is the effect it has on the gastrointestinal tract. Its history as a digestive for indigestion and flatulence is long. The Egyptians, Romans, and ancient Chinese all used it, and the Greek Dioscorides prescribed it so frequently that it came to be known as "the herb of Dioscorides." Modern science supports its use: dill is now known to inhibit the growth of *E. coli* bacteria. The German Commission E includes it on its approved list for dyspepsia. Because dill contains mineral salts, it's a good salt substitute.

It's comforting to know that a plant that adds so much flavor to food is good for you, too. There's nothing quite like dill for fish cookery, pickles, and potato salad, but my favorite use of this annual herb is in a less likely combination—with carrots in a chilled soup (A. Brockie Stevenson's Dilled, Chilled Carrot Soup, page 42).

In the garden, dill goes to seed rather quickly. To have a steady supply, you have to keep planting it. Sow seeds where they are to grow in moist, fertile, slightly acid soil in early spring and repeat at two- to three-week intervals to keep it coming.

Site it on the north side of shorter plants because it will reach five feet tall. Or try the variety 'Fernleaf,' which grows only eighteen inches tall. It's a good choice for a sunny windowsill garden.

Mrs. Adams's Salt Method for Preserving Dill

Mrs. Adams is the mother of the curator of the National Herb Garden.

1. In a widemouthed jar or plastic food container, alternate layers of kosher salt and fresh, dry dill leaves.
2. Cover with a plastic lid and store in the refrigerator.
3. Rinse off the dill with water when you are ready to use it, to get rid of the salty taste.
4. Use the dill-flavored salt for cooking.

> **TIP**
>
> *Crush dill seeds to release volatile oil before using.*

Tomato, Red Onion, and Dill Salad Bella Luna

Horst Pfeifer, whose New Orleans restaurant Bella Luna is noted for the creative use of fresh herbs, can be seen every morning riding his bicycle to the Ursuline Convent Garden, where he gardens and harvests herbs. As he weeded and harvested some beautiful dill, he tossed off this idea for a salad.

    2 ripe tomatoes, sliced
    1 large red onion, sliced thin
    ¼ cup fresh, chopped dill
    ½ cup olive oil
    2 tablespoons red wine vinegar
    ½ teaspoon salt, or to taste
      Pepper

1. Layer the tomatoes, onion, and dill in a bowl.
2. Mix together the olive oil, wine vinegar, salt, and pepper.
3. Drizzle the olive oil mixture over the vegetables.

YIELD: 3 to 4 servings

Dill Hummus

This is one of those recipes, thrown together in a few minutes, in which a cook adds an atypical ingredient and instantly regrets it. In this case, the ingredient was some beautiful dill from the garden. I had houseguests, and nothing to serve before dinner. The pantry yielded a single can of chickpeas. I decided upon hummus, remembered the beautiful dill, and threw it in before I had thought it through. I regretted it—until I tasted the hummus. This hummus does not contain tahini (sesame seed paste), but I like it this way.

    1 can (15 ounces) chickpeas, drained
    ½ cup plus 1 tablespoon olive oil

2 tablespoons lemon juice

1–2 cloves garlic, roughly chopped

2 tablespoons fresh, chopped dill

¼ teaspoon salt, or to taste

Pepper

1. Put all the ingredients into a blender.
2. Blend until smooth.
3. Adjust seasoning if necessary.

YIELD: 1¾ cups

Echinacea

ECHINACEA SPP.

BOTANICAL NAME: *Echinacea purpurea,* Asteraceae.

COMMON NAME: Coneflower.

DESCRIPTION: Perennial.

Height: To 4 feet.

Flowers: Rose-pink daisy-like flowers around a prominent central cone.

Leaves: Dark green, leathery, on strong, erect stems.

HARVEST: Dig roots in fall; harvest leaves and flowers in summer.

CULTURE: Zones 3 to 9. Grow in full sun in most any garden soil.

USE: An immune-system stimulant.

COMMENTS: Coneflowers are a wonderful addition to a perennial border and a long-lasting cut flower.

OTHER CULTIVARS AND SPECIES: *E. purpurea* 'White Swan,' 'Magnus,' 'Bright Star,' 'Kim's Kneehigh'; pale coneflower *(E. pallida)*; *E. angustifolia*; *E. tenneseensis*; *E. paradoxa.*

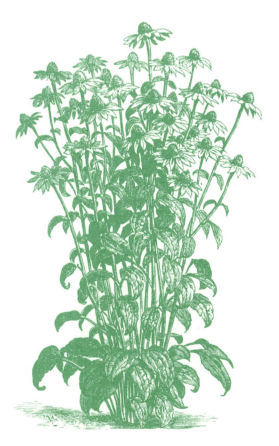

*M*ost people are surprised to learn that echinacea, the powerful herbal cure, is none other than coneflower, a beautiful native perennial. Before I began to think of it medicinally, I grew echinacea for the big, rose-pink daisy-like flowers that bloom lustily for weeks in the hottest part of the summer. In arrangements, coneflowers last so long that you are likely to throw away all of the other components before they even begin to fade.

In the garden, coneflowers attract wildlife. In midsummer, butterflies circling a patch of blooms always remind me of one of those perpetual-motion mobiles. After the flowers fade, birds flock for the seed.

If you start coneflowers from seed in the early spring, the plants will bloom modestly in the first year. These undemanding plants flower best in full sun, where, by the second year, they produce abundant bouquets—the more you pick, the more flowers appear. And the plants multiply freely by both roots and seedlings, providing a steady supply of roots for medicinal use.

Native Americans and early settlers used *Echinacea purpurea* as well as two other native species, *Echinacea pallida* and *Echinacea angustifolia*, as cure-alls. Some people think that *E. pallida* and *E. angustifolia* are more suitable for medicinal use than *E. purpurea*, but they are mistaken. All three are potent remedies. Grow the one that performs best in your garden.

All echinaceas have antiviral, antifungal, and antibacterial effects and are useful in treating colds, flu, bronchitis, and yeast and urinary tract infections. Poultices of the plant can be applied externally to poorly healing wounds.

All parts of the plant are useful. At flowering, the entire plant can be cut and dried for infusions. However, because it is so handsome, I'd rather wait until fall when I divide plants and use the roots of unwanted plants.

In the United States echinacea use dropped with the introduction of antibiotics in the early twentieth century. Only in the last decade has echinacea enjoyed a resurgence of popularity by way of Europe. In Germany, where herbal medicine has remained generally more popular and accepted, echinacea has been thoroughly researched and shown to stimulate the immune system by stimulating production of infection-fighting T cells and mimicking the action of the body's virus-fighting substance, interferon. It is on the approved list of the German Commission E.

Preparing Echinacea Roots for Storage

1. After the plants flower, divide them, replanting young divisions and reserving the oldest roots for tea.
2. Clean the roots thoroughly.
3. Chop them into small (½-inch) pieces and spread the pieces out on a plate, screen, or colander to dry. Set them in an airy, warm place out of the sun for a day or two.
4. When they are thoroughly dry, store them in a cool, dark place in a covered container. They will keep for about a year.

Echinacea Root Tea

1. Bring 2 cups water to a boil.
2. Add 1 tablespoon dried chopped echinacea root.
3. Turn down the heat, cover, and let simmer one hour (liquid should reduce by about ½ cup).
4. Strain into a container. Drink ½ cup three times a day.

Elderberry

BOTANICAL NAME: *Sambucus canadensis,* Caprifoliacae.

COMMON NAMES: Elderberry, elder.

DESCRIPTION: Deciduous shrub.

> *Height:* To 12 feet.
>
> *Flowers:* Edible, creamy-white in summer.
>
> *Leaves:* Toxic, compound.

HARVEST: Flowers when freshly opened; fruits when purple-black and fully ripe.

CULTURE: Zones 3 to 10. Moist, fertile soil, sun. Plant two shrubs for cross-pollination.

USE: For flu, colds, and fevers.

COMMENTS: Only ripe fruits and flowers are edible; leaves and stems are poisonous. Birds love the fruits.

OTHER SPECIES: European elder *(Sambucus nigra).*

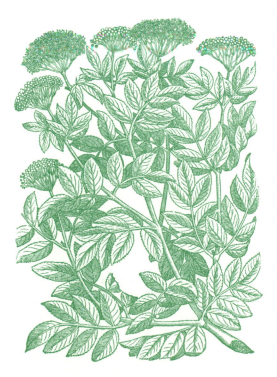

*I*n my grandmother's day, everyone seemed to have an elderberry bush *(Sambucus canadensis)* growing in the yard. Elderberries, which are native shrubs, grew just about anywhere in the country. Unfussy about soil, they would grow in acid or alkaline conditions, tolerating drought and extremes of hot and cold.

The flowers were made into fritters and the purple-black, late-summer berries into jam and wine. But when my grandmother's generation sold the houses with porches and deep yards and carriage-houses-turned-garages and moved to Florida, elderberries disappeared from the landscape. With them went the fritters, the jam, and the wine.

Now an Israeli scientist has patented Sambucol, a drug that is effective in treating flu and other viruses and that contains European elder *(Sambucus nigra)* as an active ingredient. The German Commission E includes elder flowers on its approved list as effective for colds. That—and the fact that Native Americans fed the berries of *Sambucus canadensis* to convalescing patients—has made me regard these old-fashioned shrubs with new eyes.

Small, bitter, and seedy, fresh elderberries require cooking. When combined with sugar and lemon juice in pies and jams, they're delicious. They are exceedingly rich in vitamin C and have considerable amounts of vitamin A and B vitamins. The old practice of serving warm elderberry wine for sore throat and flu not only makes sense, it seems a pleasant way to remedy the unpleasantness of illness.

For flowers and berries, you need two elderberry bushes to cross-pollinate. Stoloniferous and thick, elderberries reach twelve feet tall when grown in moist, fertile soil. If unchecked, their suckers can turn them into thickets. However, late-fall or early-winter pruning can keep them in line. They bloom on new wood. On the positive side, medicinal properties in a nourishing fruit that virtually anybody with a bit of sun in Zones 3 to 10 can grow is a real plus.

Elderberry Cordial (Nonalcoholic)

Many years ago, my sister-in-law, Kris Talley, gave me a copy of The Country Housewife's Handbook, *published by the West Kent Federation of Women's Institutes. It's chock-full of information that I've never seen elsewhere: how to cook a tough chicken, how to espalier a medlar, how to rear ducks. Its collection of old-fashioned recipes inspired this adaptation, "excellent for a cold."*

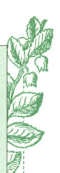
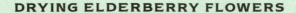

2 cups elderberries

½ cup brown sugar

½ cup sugar

4 cloves

   2-inch piece of ginger, peeled and cut into chunks

   Juice of one lemon

1. Put the berries in a mason jar and set it into a pot of water.
2. Bring the water to a boil, then simmer for about ½ hour.
3. Strain the berries and measure the juice. Discard the skins and seeds.
4. To 1 cup of the juice, add the sugars, cloves, ginger, and lemon juice and simmer for 1 hour. Cool, strain, bottle, and refrigerate.
5. To serve, add a tablespoonful to a cup of hot water.

YIELD: 1 cup syrup

Elderberry Flowers Tempura

The recipes I found for elderberry fritters were flour based and, to my mind, heavy and lumpy. Then I tried a box of prepared tempura batter and found the results far more delicate. It didn't turn the lacy flowers to lumps. I've tried other flowers that bloom at the same time—bee balm, thyme, chamomile, nasturtium—but found only the nasturtium to my liking. Elderberry flowers are superb done this way. You can break each one into four or five smaller pieces or fry the flower whole.

Vegetable oil, enough to fill a saucepan 2 inches deep
Tempura batter mix (packaged)
Elderberry flowers, 2–3 whole flowers per person

1. Heat the oil to 350°.
2. Follow the directions for mixing the tempura batter. They may not be complete. The box I bought was a sketchy translation that didn't specify the quantity of mix to add to the water. Try equal quantities of water and mix for a batter that resembles a crêpe batter.
3. Coat each flower with tempura batter and fry until golden, turning once. Drain on paper towels. Serve immediately.

Elecampane

INULA HELENIUM

BOTANICAL NAME: *Inula helenium,* Asteraceae.

COMMON NAME: Elecampane.

DESCRIPTION: Perennial.

> *Height:* To 5 feet.
>
> *Flowers:* Yellow with threadlike petals.
>
> *Leaves:* Large, coarse, to 1 foot.

HARVEST: Dig roots in fall.

CULTURE: Zones 5 to 8. Plant elecampane in rich, moist soil in sun to part shade; in Zone 7, cut it back to the ground after flowering.

USE: Immune system stimulant; effective for bacterial and fungal infections.

COMMENTS: A striking perennial.

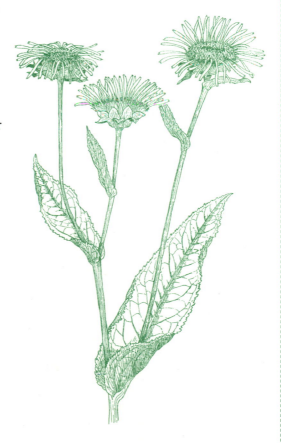

Like echinacea, elecampane first came into my garden as an ornamental, grown as much for its tall, bold foliage as for its bright yellow flowers. I started it early, from seed, on a windowsill, and it grew easily. By August its bright green, textured leaves measured over a foot in length, but the flowers—daisy-like with fine, spidery petals—didn't appear until the second season. Once you have plants, it is faster to propagate by division.

In the garden elecampane prefers a well-drained place with at least four hours of sunshine each day and resents transplanting. It is hardy in Zones 3 to 8. Growing four to five feet high, it is a great background plant in a perennial border, and the flowers are pretty in bouquets.

One of the classic medicinals, elecampane is named for Helen of Troy. Legend has it that she was gathering it when Paris abducted her—an event that launched a thousand ships. Throughout history, the roots of elecampane plants two years old and older have been used as a remedy for coughs, asthma, and indigestion. Used in Chinese, Ayurvedic, and veterinary medicine, elecampane stimulates the immune system. It is antibacterial and antifungal, it kills intestinal parasites, and it is even reputed to kill the tuberculosis bacillus. The root is a rich source of inulin, a sugar substitute for diabetics.

The bitter-tasting root may be eaten dried or cooked, but a more palatable method is to candy it by boiling it in sugar syrup.

$\mathcal{E}$lecampane Cordial

If you aren't feeling well, there's no reason to make matters worse by taking bitter medicine. Years ago, on a cold winter's night in Germany when I was coming down with a cold, I drank some Gluhwein, *a hot spiced wine, and felt much better. You can drink this elecampane cordial hot or cold. It's a good-for-what-ails-you tonic to be sipped in front of the fire on a cold winter's night.*

    1¼ cups water
      1 cup sugar
      4 ounces (about ⅔ cup) dried, chopped elecampane root
      2 cups port wine

1. Make a sugar syrup with the water and sugar.
2. When it is clear, add the elecampane root and lower the heat to a slow simmer. Simmer 10 minutes, then let the mixture cool to room temperature.
3. Strain into a large jar. Add the wine. Mix and hoard as a remedy for colds and flu.

Epazote

CHENOPODIUM AMBROSIOIDES

BOTANICAL NAME: *Chenopodium ambrosioides,* Chenopodiaceae.

COMMON NAMES: Epazote, wormseed.

DESCRIPTION: Perennial, grow as an annual in colder climates (Zone 7 and colder).

> *Height:* To 18+ inches.

> *Flowers:* Small, inconspicuous, go quickly to seed.

> *Leaves:* Narrow, rank-smelling.

HARVEST: Leaves as needed during the growing season. Cut plants as flowering begins for drying.

CULTURE: Zones 8 to 10. Sun, ordinary soil. Self-sows abundantly.

USE: A vermifuge. Add to bean dishes to prevent flatulence. Contributes a unique and authentic flavor to some Mexican dishes.

COMMENTS: You need only one plant.

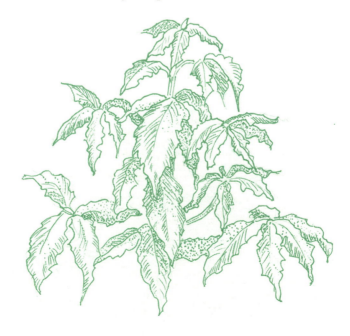

*F*amed for its antiflatulence properties, epazote has an acrid taste, essential in the complex mix of earthy, smoky flavors of traditional Mexican cuisine. Diana Kennedy, doyenne of Mexican cookery, calls it the sine qua non for the cooking of black beans. In parts of Mexico and Guatemala, no self-respecting cook would prepare a bean dish without adding it.

Its use varies by locality. In the southern part of Mexico, the fresh green leaves of epazote are chopped and added to soups and corn, bean, and fish dishes, as well as to moles and tomatillo sauces. In the north of Mexico, epazote is also used dried. Fresh, a typical sprig, perhaps a foot in length, is the equivalent of a teaspoonful of the dried leaves.

Plants grow quickly from seed. Start them indoors or sow directly in the garden after the soil has warmed. More than likely, epazote will self-sow and naturalize. Unless you operate a Mexican restaurant (and perhaps even then), you need only one plant, because epazote grows bushy and dense. Cut it back and it will send out a second and even a third crop of leaves in a single season.

Epazote has a smell as distinctive as that of cilantro, but far less pleasant. Wet ferret comes to mind. Nevertheless, when I read in Madelene Hill and Gwen Barclay's excellent *Southern Herb Growing* that epazote dried is "an effective room freshener," I tried it. And it is. Drying transforms epazote's rank odor into something far more refined and medicinal. Mixed with equal parts of mugwort *(Artemisia vulgaris)*, epazote serves as a first-rate room freshener that gives off a clean, rather neutral scent, like the faintest whiff of mown hay. I prefer this to overbearing, flowery potpourris.

Epazote has medicinal uses. It is a vermifuge—a destroyer of intestinal worms and parasites—when the leaves are made into a tea. One variety, *Chenopodium ambrosioides* var. *anthelminticum,* is especially efficacious. It is also used to deter ants. Try spreading crushed leaves in their path and see what happens.

Juan's Sopa de Albóndiga
(Meatball Soup)

Julian's Mexican Café in Santa Barbara, California, is justly famous for its authentic Mexican cuisine. Chef Juan Rodriguez shared this delectable soup flavored with fresh epazote.

2 pounds ground beef

5 ounces long-grain rice

2 eggs

2 teaspoons minced fresh epazote plus additional for garnish

1 teaspoon cumin

1 teaspoon salt

Pinch of pepper

1½ quarts boiling water

1 cup chopped carrots

1 cup chopped zucchini

1 cup chopped celery

1 large yellow onion, chopped into small-to-medium-size pieces

2 large tomatoes, chopped into small-to-medium-size pieces

1 soupspoon chicken base

1 tablespoon vegetable oil

1. Place the ground beef in a large bowl. Add the rice, eggs, epazote, cumin, salt, and pepper. Mix by hand.
2. Shape into small balls and place them in the boiling water. Cook for 20 to 25 minutes.
3. Add the chopped carrots to the meatballs and continue to cook for 5 minutes. Then add the zucchini and celery and continue to cook.
4. Meanwhile, pan-sauté the yellow onion, tomato, and chicken base in the vegetable oil until the onion is brown. Add to the soup.
5. When serving this wonderful soup, add a small pinch of epazote to each bowl.

YIELD: 12 to 16 servings

Sopa de Setas (Wild Mushroom Soup)

After she described this soup to me, Nicki Zuchowicz got no rest. I pestered her to pester her father, Simon, in Mexico for the recipe. It was months in coming, but worth the wait because it is every bit as good as she remembered. Assortments of wild mushrooms including oysters and criminis are sometimes available at supermarkets.

10–12 ounces assorted wild mushrooms (not brown, or portobellos)
1 chopped onion
3 cloves garlic, chopped
2 ounces butter
½ teaspoon salt
   Ground black pepper
2 cups chicken broth
3 sprigs epazote (or 1 teaspoon dry, rubbed through a sieve to eliminate stems and veins)

1. Wash and dry the mushrooms and cut them into small strips. Set aside.
2. Fry the onion and garlic in the butter for 5 minutes, then add half the mushrooms. Fry very slowly for another 10 minutes.
3. Blend the remaining mushrooms with the chicken broth and the epazote.
4. Add the blended mushrooms to the pot with salt and ground black pepper. Cook over low heat until tender.

YIELD: 4 servings

Epazote-Artemisia Room Freshener

If you'd like an air freshener that doesn't smell like powder room potpourris, try this one. Not cloying, it freshens without announcing itself.

2–3 cups dried epazote leaves
   2 cups dried artemisia leaves

Mix leaves together and place in a widemouthed bowl.

Epazote Butter

¼ pound butter, softened
  1 tablespoon fresh epazote, chopped

Combine the butter and the epazote in a mortar and blend with a pestle. Serve with corn on the cob or melted over corn.

Fava Beans

VICIA FABA

BOTANICAL NAME: *Vicia faba,* Leguminosae.

COMMON NAMES: Fava beans, broad beans.

DESCRIPTION: Annual vegetable.

> *Height:* To 4 feet.
>
> *Flowers:* White pea flowers with distinctive black markings.
>
> *Leaves:* Light green, on lax stems that need support.

HARVEST: When pods droop, shell and eat fresh, or dry beans for storage.

CULTURE: Start favas early in rich, moist soil; provide support for stems as for peas. Companionable favas grow favorably with members of the cabbage family.

USE: A delicious way to add L-dopa to the diet.

COMMENTS: Some people of Mediterranean origin are allergic to fava beans.

Viagra, eat your heart out!
  —Dr. James Duke

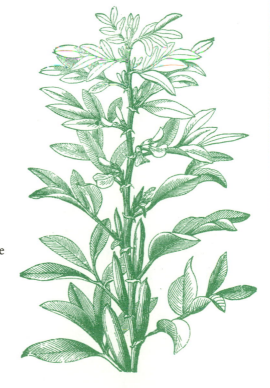

When I first heard how fava or broad beans contain more L-dopa, a compound that helps men achieve erections, than any other food, I was curious. When I read that these beans have a well-deserved reputation as aphrodisiacs, I ordered seeds—many more than I needed so that I might sprout some—and I bought some dried favas to try cooking before my harvest came in. Everything I subsequently learned about favas came the hard way.

It would seem that, as one of the oldest foods in the world and one of the most nutritious, they would be easy to come by and easier still to grow. Not so. Not every seed catalog carries them (see Sources).

Once you find varieties of fava beans such as 'Broad Windsor' in a specialty seed catalog, their journey from seed to table is still not down-hill, especially if you live in an area of hot summers. Like peas, fava beans are a cool-weather crop. Unlike peas, they require a rather long growing season—about ninety days. This makes it difficult, but not im-possible, to squeak them in between the last blasts of winter and the first truly hot weather in summer. Gardeners living in the Gulf Coast states can plant favas as a winter crop. The fresh beans are a real treat.

Nora's Fava Bean Succotash

From the kitchen of Washington's wonderful Restaurant Nora, this recipe can be made either from dried fava beans that have been soaked, deskinned, and cooked, or from fresh ones—a wonderful early-summer treat.

2 tablespoons olive oil
½ cup fresh, young fava beans, removed from their pods (or
    ½ cup cooked dried fava beans)
1 cup fresh corn kernels
1 tomato, chopped
    Salt and freshly ground black pepper

1. Heat the olive oil in a skillet over a medium heat.
2. Add the young, fresh fava beans (or cooked fava beans, if using dried) and sauté for 2 minutes.

3. Add the corn and sauté for a further 2 minutes.
4. Add the chopped tomato, season, and combine well. Serve immediately.

YIELD: 4 servings

TIP

You can buy dried fava beans. If possible, buy them already skinned. Otherwise, you will have to remove their skins after soaking them, a laborious process.

Fennel

FOENICULUM VULGARE SYN. *F. OFFICINALE*

BOTANICAL NAME: *Foeniculum vulgare,* Apiaceae.

COMMON NAMES: Fennel, tea fennel.

DESCRIPTION: Short-lived perennial.

Height: To 6 feet.

Flowers: Yellow in umbels; turn toward the sun.

Leaves: Fine, bright green (or bronze or burgundy); form "clouds" of foliage.

HARVEST: The leaves as needed to season fish, the seeds as umbels begin to turn brown; hang the umbels up to dry before storing the seeds.

CULTURE: Grow fennel in near neutral, rich, moist, loose loam; cut the seeds off before they fall. Taprooted fennel may seed prolifically in the garden and is hard to weed out.

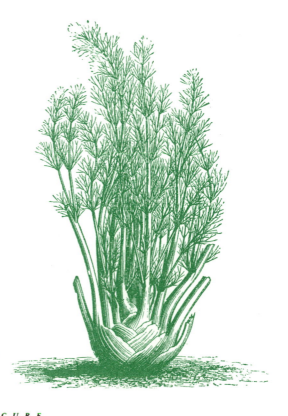

USE: A proven digestive, for flatulence.

COMMENTS: Fennel oil should not be given to pregnant women. People with sensitive stomachs may not tolerate raw fennel or its herbal supplements. Anyone harvesting fennel from the wild should make certain that the plant they plan to eat is fennel and not poison hemlock, a look-alike.

OTHER VARIETY: Florence fennel, or *finocchio (Foeniculum vulgare* var. *azoricum)*.

Above the lower plants it towers,
The Fennel with its yellow flowers;
And in an earlier age than ours,
Was gifted with wondrous powers,
Lost vision to restore.
—Longfellow

Not all of the curative properties traditionally assigned to fennel are confirmed by modern science. Fennel won't restore lost vision and it won't keep witches away. However, its history as a digestive is long and stands up to modern scrutiny. Have you ever noticed the bowls of fennel seeds in Indian restaurants? They are there to aid customers' digestion. Compounds in the seeds help to relieve flatulence.

One of the ways in which the ancient Greeks used fennel is also supported by scientific study. The Greeks used fennel to stimulate nursing mothers' production of milk. It is now known that fennel has a mild estrogenic effect. For this reason, people with estrogen-dependent breast tumors should not eat fennel until more study has been done.

Fennel comes in many forms, including red and burgundy varieties and a lovely bronze, reputed to be somewhat hardier.

Fennel has naturalized along the Pacific Coast—notably near the Big Sur area. However, I would strongly advise against harvesting fennel from the wild. One plant that looks like fennel but does not have its characteristic anise scent is poison hemlock.

Fennel, *Foeniculum vulgare,* is a tall plant with clouds of feathery, soft green leaves, or fronds, that impart an anise flavor to fish cookery. Perennial and probably hardy to Zone 6, fennel is most often grown as an annual in the herb or vegetable garden, where it often self-sows in the rich, loose, moist soil it favors. The ribbed stems resemble a big-boned, lanky celery that broadens at the base as the season progresses. These stems may be eaten, but generally speaking this fennel is grown for its seeds.

Following umbels of yellow flowers that reveal kinship to carrots, dill, and Queen Anne's lace, fennel seeds appear in late August. They are used to flavor sausages, and, crushed, for a digestive tea. Fennel seeds are on the German Commission E's approved list for alleviating upper respiratory catarrh and dyspepsia.

Florence fennel (*Foeniculum vulgare* var. *azoricum*), also called *finocchio*, is an annual form of fennel, grown primarily for its edible, mildly anise-flavored bulbous base. This fennel's more substantial stems lend themselves to use as a vegetable. Shorter than its perennial relative, Florence fennel usually grows only two feet tall. It, too, produces seeds for flavoring. Delicious eaten raw in salads, Florence fennel is great braised in chicken broth, grilled, or stewed.

It is easy to grow fennel from seed sown in early spring where the plant is to grow. If you are growing it for the greens only, start new seeds every two weeks. Choose a site in full sun with fairly rich, neutral soil that has good drainage.

Florence fennel demands a soil that has been enriched with compost or manure. It prefers cool growing conditions, but it needs a full three months to develop bulbs. Start it in early summer and give it plenty of water to help it through the heat. Otherwise the plant will bolt, sending up flowers and seeds before the bulbs form. The variety 'Zefa Fino' is reputed to be bolt resistant.

To preserve the delicate anise flavor, blanch stems by hilling up the soil around the base when Florence fennel stalks stand a foot tall. Harvest when the bulbs are about three inches in diameter.

Thinly sliced Florence fennel is a classic ingredient on an antipasto platter and is equally good in salads. An easy way to cook Florence fennel is to blanch stalks for five minutes in chicken stock, then drain and broil them, topped with Parmesan and chopped oregano. Or add chopped stalks to soups, sauces, stews, and roasted vegetables for a bright anise flavor.

Herbes de Provence

A blend frequently used in the South of France, herbes de Provence may include a number of herbs. Its distinctive flavor, however, comes from the fennel and lavender.

    3 tablespoons dried marjoram
    3 tablespoons dried thyme
    2 tablespoons dried summer savory
 1½ teaspoons dried rosemary
    ½ teaspoon fennel seeds
    ¼ teaspoon dried lavender flowers
    ½ teaspoon dried sage
    ½ teaspoon dried mint

Mix all the ingredients together. Use for seasoning veal, pork, or turkey.

YIELD: ⅓ cup

Fennel, Orange, and Cabbage Salad

Barbara Pratt shared this hearty salad, which blends the contrasting tastes of Florence fennel, peppers, oranges, and bacon. Take care to cut the ingredients into pieces of a manageable size.

    2 large fennel bulbs, sliced into fine strips lengthwise, with core
       removed
    1 tablespoon minced fennel tops
    1 small red pepper, cut into fine strips
    1 small green pepper, cut into fine strips
    1 small hot chili pepper, seeded and minced
    2 oranges, peeled, sectioned, and seeded
    3 tablespoons olive oil
    ¼ pound bacon, cut into 2-inch pieces

1 small onion, thinly sliced
1 cup finely shredded green cabbage
¾ cup white wine vinegar
    Salt
¼ teaspoon ground black pepper
1 teaspoon lime juice

1. Combine the sliced fennel, fennel tops, peppers, and orange sections and set aside.
2. Put 2 tablespoons of the oil in a 12-inch skillet and cook the bacon and the onion over medium heat.
3. With a slotted spoon, remove the onion when it is golden, then the bacon when it is browned. Set aside.
4. Cook the cabbage in the remaining oil over medium-high heat until it is tender-crisp.
5. Add the cabbage, bacon, onion, vinegar, salt, and pepper to the fennel mixture. Toss to coat well.
6. Sprinkle with the lime juice before serving.

YIELD: 8 servings

Terry Pogue's Fennel and Apple Salad

Terry Pogue, who hosted the Washington, D.C., radio show Plant Talk, *is also renowned as an elegant hostess. She shared this unusual recipe with me. The paper-thin slices that give this salad its delicacy can be made with a mandoline (I have an inexpensive one and it works fine). If you don't have a mandoline, slice the fennel and apple as thin as is humanly possible. The original recipe calls for 15 juniper berries instead of cranberries. You can buy juniper berries or pick and dry your own.*

1 bulb Florence fennel
1 Granny Smith apple
1 teaspoon lemon juice
¼ cup dried cranberries, or 15 juniper berries

2 tablespoons olive oil
  Salt
  Freshly ground pepper

1. Trim the fennel, and then cut it in half through the core, keeping some of the feathery fronds for garnish.
2. Cut the apple into quarters and core it, but do not peel it.
3. Using a mandoline, cut the fennel against the grain as thinly as possible.
4. Also using the mandoline, cut the apple into the thinnest possible slices.
5. In a nonreactive bowl, toss together the fennel, apple, lemon juice, cranberries, and olive oil. Season to taste with salt and pepper. (Or, if omitting the cranberries and adding juniper, crush the juniper berries with the side of a knife, and then mince. Stir them into the salad, toss, and let sit for 5 minutes before serving.)
6. Just before serving, garnish with the minced feathery fennel tops.

YIELD: 4 servings

Feverfew

TANACETUM PARTHENIUM

BOTANICAL NAME: *Tanacetum parthenium,* Asteraceae.

COMMON NAME: Feverfew.

DESCRIPTION: Perennial.

Height: To 4 feet.

Flowers: Small daisy-like flowers, white with golden centers.

Leaves: Light green, cut edges.

HARVEST: Cut fresh leaves as needed.

CULTURE: Site feverfew in sun to part shade. It tolerates poor soil and needs excellent drainage. It self-sows happily in most gardens.

USE: For migraines, inflammation.

COMMENTS: Feverfew's effects are cumulative.

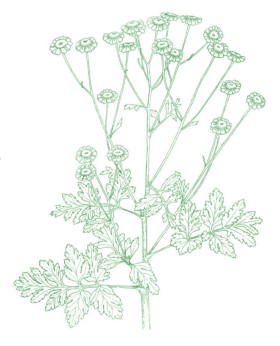

*F*everfew made a big splash in the 1970s when English researchers found that it cured some migraine sufferers completely and significantly reduced the incidence of migraine headaches in other people. The dose was between one and four leaves each day and the effects were cumulative.

If you are in the throes of a migraine, eating feverfew leaves won't cure it. You have to eat them as a preventive herbal remedy for at least a month.

Although I no longer have migraines, I remember in excruciating detail the five or six I experienced. If I ever got them again, I would certainly eat feverfew in place of lettuce on my sandwiches, no matter how bitter the leaves. (And I would hope I was not among the small percentage of people who get mouth ulcers from eating raw feverfew.)

The active agent in feverfew is parthenolide. It is thought to work by dilating cerebral blood vessels, so the kinds of migraines it would help are those involving constriction of those vessels. However, the prestigious British medical journal *The Lancet* has reported that feverfew inhibits the agents that cause inflammation in migraines and arthritis better than aspirin. In short, it's worth a try, no matter what the cause of the migraine.

Feverfew is one of many herbs described in the first century A.D. by Dioscorides, reputed to have been a Greek physician with the Roman army. He prescribed it for melancholia. This use finds validation today. In *The Green Pharmacy*, Dr. Jim Duke writes that long-term feverfew users may experience a "mild tranquilizing or sedative effect."

Throughout history, feverfew has been used in much the same way aspirin is today. In his 1640 work *Theatrum Botanicum*, London herbalist John Parkinson recommends feverfew for "all paines in the head." Feverfew has been given to induce restful sleep, for cramps, for relief from arthritis, and as a mild sedative (when given as an infusion).

Tincture of feverfew is readily available in health food stores, but plants and seeds are also easy to come by. Start seeds indoors to transplant outside when the weather is settled. Easy to grow, feverfew is a short-lived perennial that grows to two or three feet tall. It will make it through the winter in Zones 3 to 9 as long as fast drainage is provided.

A handsome plant with pretty, light green, deeply lobed leaves, feverfew bears clusters of small white flowers with golden centers; the flowers look like tiny daisies. The flowers may be dried for winter bouquets. There are double forms available, as well as plants with golden foliage.

Feverfew-Cucumber Sandwich

This recipe originated in a search for a civilized way for migraine sufferers to in-gest fresh feverfew. More than merely civilized, this delicate tea sandwich turned out to be delicious.

⅓–½ cucumber, peeled and sliced very thin
2 feverfew leaves, chopped fine
2 teaspoons cream
Salt and pepper
Butter
2 thin slices of bread

1. Place the cucumber slices in a bowl.
2. Top with the chopped feverfew leaves.
3. Pour the cream over the cucumber and feverfew. Add salt and pep-per. Allow to stand at least 30 minutes.
4. Thinly butter the slices of bread. Cover one with the cucumber slices (the feverfew bits will cling) and top with the second slice.

YIELD: 1 sandwich

Feverfew Tea

1. Boil 10 ounces of water.
2. Steep 4 grams of dried feverfew (about a heaping teaspoon) for 5 to 10 minutes in the water when it has just boiled.
3. Strain and drink.

Garlic

ALLIUM SATIVUM

BOTANICAL NAME: *Allium sativum,* Liliaceae.

COMMON NAME: Garlic.

DESCRIPTION: Bulbous perennial.

Height: To 3 feet.

Flowers: White. Cut these off to strengthen the bulbs.

Leaves: Long, narrow; can be cut and sliced into salads and soups.

HARVEST: Wait until the foliage turns yellow and the plants stop growing; dig the bulbs carefully to avoid damaging them.

CULTURE: Zones 3 to 9. Garlic thrives in soil enriched with a balanced fertilizer; raised beds provide the best drainage. Keep well weeded. Garlic is rarely bothered by pests other than weeds; it discourages pests around beets, lettuce, and roses.

USE: Garlic is an antiviral, antibacterial, antifungal food that lowers cholesterol and blood pressure and improves circulation.

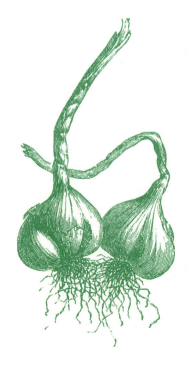

COMMENTS: Raw garlic is thought to have the greatest medicinal benefits.

OTHER SPECIES: Elephant garlic, or wild leek *(Allium ampeloprasum),* needs deeper planting (4 to 6 inches) but has the same growth requirements and a milder flavor.

Folks constantly ask about the "secret" that has kept us alive so long. . . . We start our day by drinking a full glass of water, followed by a teaspoon of cod liver oil and a whole clove of garlic. A whole, raw clove—that's right. . . . We chop the clove as finely as we can, then scoop it up with a spoon, and swallow it all at once, without chewing, to prevent odor.

—Bessie Delany, centenarian,
The Delany Sisters' Book of Everyday Wisdom

*F*or as long as there has been written history, there has been documentation of garlic's medicinal use. Over two thousand years ago, an unknown hand incised a prescription containing garlic into the moist clay of a Sumerian tablet. Along with gold and oil, garlic was among the provisions stored in King Tut's tomb for his journey into the afterlife. And it was garlic that fortified Ulysses against Circe. Hippocrates, Dioscorides, and Pliny all recommended it for a variety of ailments—including leprosy and cancer, for which it is still used in Ayurvedic medicine. Called "Russian penicillin" for its use in treating wounded soldiers in World War II, fresh garlic is a potent antibiotic.

"Garlic is emerging as an alternative to prescription antibiotics," say the editors of *Herbs for Health*, a well-respected magazine, adding that because some bacteria become resistant to prescription antibiotics, a naturally occurring, less specifically targeted remedy such as garlic is all the more valuable.

Today there is plenty of research being undertaken on garlic. The more research that is conducted, the more garlic's medicinal reputation is substantiated. Garlic has killed cancer cells in test tubes and lowered cholesterol. Both an ancient remedy and a modern cure, it is an antiviral food that also lowers blood pressure. And it improves circulation—a clue to its reputation as an aphrodisiac. Garlic is included on the German Commission E's approved list as a preventive measure for age-dependent vascular changes.

Some studies indicate that the incidence of cancer drops among those who consume garlic regularly. Recent research suggests it can cut the risk of preeclampsia in pregnancy and inhibit cancer-causing agents from binding to human breast cells. The presence of compounds such as quercetin that retard inflammation may make garlic useful in the treatment of allergies.

According to Dr. Michael T. Murray, a naturopathic physician who writes extensively on herbal medicine, the daily dose of garlic needed to obtain health benefits is "a total allicin potential of 4,000 mcg . . . roughly one to four cloves of fresh garlic."

Some experts think that when garlic is cooked or dried, it loses some of its health benefits. Others think that it is only allicin that decreases with cooking or drying and that there are other beneficial compounds in garlic that have not yet been identified. One study suggested that crushing the garlic and then allowing it to rest for ten minutes before cooking increased its cancer-resisting ability over garlic that was crushed and cooked immediately.

In any case, cooked garlic loses none of its value in flavoring foods. For best results, use it frequently any way you can. Raw garlic is delicious in salad dressings and cold soups such as gazpacho.

There are virtually dozens of strains of garlic, and they all respond differently to local growing conditions. Try several to see which grows best for you. Stiffneck (*Allium sativum* var. *ophioscorodon*) types develop a row of cloves around a rather large, stiff central neck. Softneck (*Allium sativum* var. *sativum*) types grow double rows of cloves and lend themselves to braiding.

When you buy garlic from a seed catalog (see Sources), what you will receive will be intact bulbs, or "heads," of garlic, often sold by weight. Each bulb will produce between eight and fifteen new bulbs. A pound of garlic—between five and ten bulbs, depending upon their size—ought to produce enough of a crop to keep you supplied through the winter. The "seeds" are the individual cloves. You will have to separate these gently. You may find that the outer cloves are plump and promising and the inner ones small and thin. Reserve the latter for use in soups and stews and set the big cloves in the ground with the pointy end up, about two inches deep and six inches apart in a place with very rich garden soil, sun, and adequate moisture.

Although garlic is rarely bothered by insect pests, cold, wet conditions can encourage molds. Raised beds ensure the good drainage garlic requires. Keep beds well weeded. According to vegetable gardening expert

Eliot Coleman, garlic should not be planted in a place where a cabbage-family crop grew previously or the yield will be lowered substantially.

The time to plant garlic is not in spring, but in fall at about the time of the first frost, four to six weeks before the ground freezes. Like the spring-flowering bulbs of tulips and daffodils, the idea is to let fall-planted garlic develop a root system but not give it enough time to send up leaves.

Keep the bed of garlic well weeded. Feed at two-week intervals with compost or cottonseed meal throughout the spring, stopping in summer when the bulbs begin to form underground.

In summer, garlic sends up flower stalks. A bed of stiffneck garlic buds on tall, twisting stems looks like a flock of geese with double-jointed necks. Unfortunately, it's best to cut the flower buds off before the stalks are a foot tall to prevent the plant from putting all of its energy into flower production. (You can grow one or two plants in the border to enjoy the flowers.) The good news is that these flowering stalks make a wonderful once-in-the-summer vegetable.

After removing the flowers, wait until the foliage yellows to stop watering the plants. Bend the tops to the ground to speed up dormancy. When there is no longer any sign of life in the tops, carefully dig up a bulb and examine it. Mature bulbs have skins around the individual cloves and papery layers around the bulb.

The next step is curing the garlic bulbs. Lay them out in a dry, shady, well-ventilated place for a week or so before removing the stems and roots and storing the bulbs. I keep them in baskets in a room that stays at about 60 degrees Fahrenheit over the winter. You can braid softneck varieties in groups of ten or so and hang them up.

In my Mid-Atlantic garden, the elephant garlic *(Allium ampelo-prasum)*, actually a garlic-flavored leek, was especially gratifying for its giant-size cloves of a delightfully mild garlic flavor. Although it weakens the cloves, I let some of the pretty white flowers grow.

Roasted Garlic and Eggplant Soup

François Dionot, founder of l'Academie de Cuisine in Bethesda, Maryland, generously shares this fantastic soup recipe. A consummate chef, he suggests floating garlic rosettes on the soup for a prettier presentation.

2 medium eggplants
1 head of garlic
   Olive oil
2 tablespoons butter
1 onion, sliced
1 leek, white part only, sliced
3 cups chicken stock
   Salt and pepper
1 cup heavy cream
   Garlic Rosettes (recipe follows), optional (prepare ahead)

1. Halve the eggplants and put them on a tray with some olive oil. Roast in a 350° oven for about 30 minutes.
2. Halve the head of garlic, place on aluminum foil, and sprinkle with olive oil. Enclose in the foil and roast along with the eggplant for 25 minutes.
3. Meanwhile, heat the butter in a large skillet. Gently sauté the onion and leek until tender.
4. When the eggplant is done, remove the meat from the skin by scraping it out with a spoon. Squeeze the garlic cloves out of their skins.
5. Add the eggplant, garlic, and chicken stock to the onion mixture. Season with salt and pepper. Cover and simmer for ½ hour.
6. Purée in a blender and add the heavy cream.
7. Garnish with Garlic Rosettes.

YIELD: 6 servings

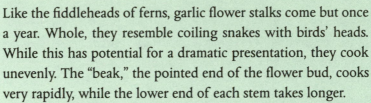

GARLIC FLOWER STALKS

Like the fiddleheads of ferns, garlic flower stalks come but once a year. Whole, they resemble coiling snakes with birds' heads. While this has potential for a dramatic presentation, they cook unevenly. The "beak," the pointed end of the flower bud, cooks very rapidly, while the lower end of each stem takes longer.

As the flower stalk matures, it becomes stiffer (and inedible). Harvest the stalks when they are thin and curled—at about 12 inches. The bottom ends of the stalks will be stiff; cut these off before cooking. Poach like beans or stir-fry.

Garlic Rosettes

These add a beautiful and flavorful finish to Roasted Garlic and Eggplant Soup (see recipe above).

1. Put equal parts garlic and softened butter into a blender with enough cream to facilitate blending.
2. Spoon the mixture into a pastry bag and, using a fluted tip, squeeze out rosettes onto a baking sheet.
3. Place in the freezer.
4. Float the rosettes on soup just before serving.

Chunky Gazpacho with Lemon Balm

Gazpacho is one of the best-tasting ways to eat raw garlic. There are many recipes for gazpacho around, and it's hard to go wrong with succulent garden tomatoes. I vary this, sometimes substituting a zucchini when I don't have a cucumber. Either way, this soup is cool and delicious with lemony, mood-lifting lemon balm.

1 cucumber, chopped
5 tomatoes, quartered

1 large onion, chopped
4 cloves garlic, peeled
6 sprigs (4–5 leaves each) of lemon balm plus 1 sprig for garnish
  Juice of 1 lime
2 tablespoons olive oil
  Chunk of French bread (or 1 slice twelve-grain bread), broken
  into small pieces

1. Put all the ingredients except the bread and 1 sprig of lemon balm
   into a blender and blend until just chunky.
2. Add the bread and blend for 10 seconds, or just long enough to
   moisten the bread and break it into smaller pieces.
3. Chill for at least 3 hours. (Store in the blender or a 1-quart container.)
4. Serve with a sprinkling of chopped lemon balm (from the remaining
   sprig).

YIELD: 4 servings

Roasted Garlic Grits

*A comfort food, grits are traditionally loaded with fat or cheese. In order to give
them a rich taste without loads of calories, I tried adding plenty of garlic and
broth. Served this way, grits are the perfect companion to roast beef, lamb, or
grilled portobello mushrooms.*

1 head of garlic
1 teaspoon olive oil
2 cups water
2 cups beef or chicken stock, or 1 can broth
1 cup instant grits
½ teaspoon salt

1. Set the head of garlic on a square of aluminum foil, drizzle it with
   the olive oil, and wrap the foil around it.
2. Roast for 25 minutes at 350°. Allow to cool.
3. Squeeze the garlic pulp into a saucepan.

4. Add the water and stock.
5. With the back of a spoon, mix the garlic into the water and stock.
6. Heat to boiling and add the instant grits and salt to the boiling liquid.
7. Cook about 5 minutes.

YIELD: 6 servings

TIP

Crushing a clove of fresh garlic with the side of a knife before chopping it is thought to release more of the beneficial compound allicin.

Ginger

ZINGIBER OFFICINALE

BOTANICAL NAME: *Zingiber officinale,* Zingiberaceae.

COMMON NAMES: Ginger, culinary ginger.

DESCRIPTION: Tender perennial.

> *Height:* To 5 feet.
>
> *Flowers:* Insignificant.
>
> *Leaves:* Bright green.

HARVEST: Cut off a small section from a growing root (actually a rhizome, called a "hand").

CULTURE: Ginger requires warmth, very rich soil, plentiful water, and full sun from Zone 6 northward. Cut back on water and allow ginger to rest over winter inside.

USE: Use ginger for nausea, for morning and motion sickness, and as a digestive.

COMMENTS: Ginger really works for nausea.

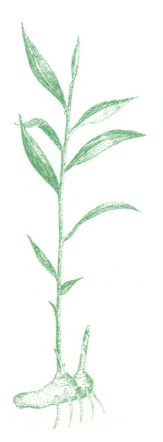

*U*nless you live in a really warm place—Zone 8 or above—ginger won't be perennial in your garden. Elsewhere, it's fun to grow ginger over the summer and harvest it before the weather turns cold.

All-around good for you, ginger contains enzymes that aid digestion and guard against flatulence. Given as a tea or candied, ginger is a safe way to treat nausea in children and morning sickness. In a study published in the

British medical journal *The Lancet* (March 1982), ginger was found to be more effective in stopping motion sickness than Dramamine. The German Commission E includes ginger on its approved list for dyspepsia and motion sickness.

Ginger's essential oils can aid in reducing fevers, relieving arthritis, and boosting the strength of the heart muscle. Ginger is also an antioxidant. It is reputed to be an aphrodisiac.

Medicinal properties aside, ginger is indispensable in the kitchen. I can't remember when I started using it, but now there are always a couple of knobby roots at hand. They disappear quickly as they get grated and chopped into soups and stir-fries. I use far too much of it to keep myself supplied, but I grow it anyway for the once-a-year thrill of superior fresh roots. Homegrown ginger is fresher than anything you can buy. The skin is very thin and the roots are juicy and far less sharp-tasting than those of the supermarket variety.

Perhaps the easiest way to get a start, if you can't find a plant of *Zingiber officinale*, is to do what I did: buy a ginger root and pot it up. If you start with what you know is culinary ginger, you'll know it's edible. Edible ginger is *Zingiber officinale*, not the same, nor as handsome, nor as readily available as some of the very ornamental gingers—usually *Hedychium* species.

Choose a root with smooth, tight skin. Barely cover the root with very rich soil. Keep it warm and keep it moist. Very soon you'll get a thin shoot with longish leaves that, unfortunately, never achieves the grace and charm of ornamental ginger. The foliage of culinary ginger looks rather like emaciated corn.

Most gingers are native to the tropical forests of Asia, where they usually grow in shade, under the tree canopy. The farther north you grow them, however, the more sun they need: full sun from Zone 6 northward.

Ginger also requires rich soil, plentiful moisture, and heat—the kind of humid, sweltering days that melt other plants. It is under these very hot conditions that ginger's roots, called "hands," fan outward in much the same manner as those of irises.

If you live in an area where the ground freezes, use the opportunity to harvest your ginger. Simply cut off the rootlets, wash off the soil, and allow them to dry with good air circulation. Pull away the young new plants that haven't yet formed tubers, pot them up, and bring them inside in the fall. Cut off the top growth and let them go dormant, giving just enough water to keep the roots from drying out. Start them up again in a sunny window in spring and transplant into the garden when the soil warms.

Mioga ginger *(Z. mioga)* is a Japanese ginger, grown not only for its root but for the yellow flowers that are served tempura-style in Japan. I grow Mioga ginger, hardier than *Z. officinale*, in Zone 7. In China its roots and leaves are used for treating malaria and insect and scorpion bites, and in a decoction for inflamed eyes.

Pommes de Marie-Eve

This recipe was going to be called "Neil Riddell's Gingered Apple Juice." Just before I asked Neil for written permission to publish it, he became engaged. His sister, Lucy, who had invented the recipe, renamed it in honor of his fiancée. She suggests cloves or a cinnamon stick for added flavor, or—for the older crowd—boosting its punch with a little whiskey.

Try this soothing hot drink the next time you have a sore throat. Delicious even with canned apple juice, it is outstanding with fresh juice. And it works!

3-inch piece unpeeled gingerroot, cut into 5–6¼-inch slices
3 cloves, optional
1 cinnamon stick, optional
10 ounces apple juice
Whiskey, optional

1. Heat the ginger slices, cloves, and cinnamon stick in the apple juice to a very slow simmer.
2. Allow to simmer for 10 to 20 minutes. Do not boil.
3. Cool and strain before drinking. If adding whiskey, do so at this point.

YIELD: 2 servings

> **TIP**
>
> *For a gas reliever, mix one teaspoon of grated fresh ginger pulp and one teaspoon of lime juice and take after eating.*
>
> *Keep a gingerroot next to the stove. Try grating it into stir-fries and dressings.*

Gingered Pear Tart

I learned to make plum tart when I lived in Germany. This version uses pears instead, for a much more subtle taste that benefits from ginger's pep. Simple and elegant, this tart is perfect all by itself, served with gingery hot tea. Extravagant people may wish to add a dollop of ice cream.

    1 cup flour
    ⅔ cup plus 2 tablespoons sugar
    4 ounces butter, softened and cut into ½-ounce pats
      Pinch of salt
    1 tablespoon grated ginger
    3 pears, peeled, cored, and cut into thin slices lengthwise

1. Preheat the oven to 375°.
2. Using knives or a pastry mixer, combine the flour, ⅔ cup of the sugar, and the butter and salt. Do not overwork the mixture or the crust will be stiff and cookie-like—not all bad, but harder to eat with a fork.
3. With a light touch, spread the dough evenly over the bottom of a springform or cake pan.
4. Sprinkle the grated ginger over the dough.
5. Arrange the pear slices, overlapping them slightly, in concentric rings, beginning at the outside and working inward.
6. Sprinkle the remaining 2 tablespoons of the sugar over the pears.
7. Bake for 25 minutes, or until the crust is browned.

YIELD: 1 tart that serves 8

Ginseng

BOTANICAL NAME: *Panax quinquefolius,* Araliaceae.

COMMON NAMES: Ginseng, seng.

DESCRIPTION: Woodland perennial.

> *Height:* To 18 inches.

> *Flowers:* Greenish white ball.

> *Leaves:* Divided into 3 to 7 leaflets.

HARVEST: Dig roots after 5 to 7 years.

CULTURE: Ginger requires shade and rich, deep, humusy soil; a mulch of shredded hardwood is helpful.

USE: As a sexual and general tonic.

COMMENTS: Large doses of ginseng are said to raise blood pressure.

OTHER SPECIES: *Panax ginseng, Panax trifolius.*

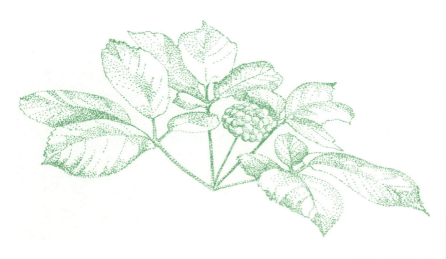

*V*olumes have been written about ginseng. No other herb under cultivation enjoys its fame and lore. In China, its reputation as an aphrodisiac and a longevity tonic goes back five thousand years. There, both the Asian species, *Panax ginseng,* and the North American species, *Panax quinquefolius,* are held in great esteem today.

It is said that one of the first diplomatic liaisons between China and the United States took place in George Washington's time, when ginseng, then a common plant in North American woodland, was exported to China.

Unfortunately, ginseng is no longer common in American woodland. Over two centuries of development and "seng" harvesters have made it rare in the wild. One small way to offset the loss of wild ginseng is to grow it in home gardens. Nursery-propagated seeds and roots are increasingly available (see Sources). Reward the people who grow ginseng ethically with your business and increase the number of ginseng plants overall. Growing your own is a very real possibility if you have the right site.

What American ginseng needs is full shade and a very cool, moist root run in deep humus. On the average residential property, these conditions are difficult to find, especially in the mid-Atlantic region and the South, where high temperatures cause the soil to dry out in summer. Because the largest commercial growers of ginseng are located in places like Wisconsin, I think that ginseng is easier to grow in a cool climate. However, its native range extends from Quebec south to Georgia and west to Oklahoma.

About eight years ago, I purchased twenty one-year-old roots. They were cream-color and about the size of my pinkie. I planted them in shady places around my garden. These dwindled to three ginseng plants. One of these is smaller—about six inches tall—than the others; this makes me think it is *Panax trifolius,* an American species also native to this area. It probably came into my garden, as either seed or small root, during a "plant save" from a construction site.

The remaining two are over a foot tall, the size that *P. quinquefolius* is supposed to be. They occupy odd places where the sun never shines, on moist slopes that are always cooler than their surroundings—the sort of corner where leaves and organic debris accumulate over winter. This spring, they produced seedlings.

James Duke, author of *The Green Pharmacy*, thinks deer eat ginseng. To protect his plants, he says, "I have antler-like branches sticking up around my ginseng plant, covered with human hair, on which I occasionally urinate."

Although I've read reports that debunk ginseng's reputation, five thousand years of tradition, along with anecdotal reports and new research, support its use as both a sexual tonic and for longevity. Ginseng is called an "adaptogen," a substance that generally strengthens the body and increases its ability to handle stresses.

Speaking at the Fourth International Herb Symposium, herbalist Ed Smith said that while ginseng is considered an aphrodisiac, it works as one mainly in the sense that it strengthens the sexual as well as other organs of the body. He cited experiments with rats that sired or bore offspring later in life when fed ginseng. Typically, he stated, the effect of ginseng can be subtle. Human subjects sometimes didn't know it was working until they stopped taking it and missed the sense of well-being it had provided.

Ginseng appears on the German Commission E's approved list. Useful as a fortification tonic and a convalescence drug, it also improves concentration.

The part of ginseng that is used medicinally is the root, generally harvested after six or seven years. Commercial ginseng is dried and powdered or used in extracts. Health food stores often carry whole roots as well. Herbalists recommend chewing on a piece of the fresh or dried root that is the size of the last digit of your little finger.

Even though there are three roots growing in my garden, the thought of digging up one of these shy, rare wildlings seems a desecration. Until I have several dozen, this is one herb I will buy from an ethical source rather than harvest for myself.

Goldenseal

BOTANICAL NAME: *Hydrastis canadensis,* Ranunculaceae.

COMMON NAMES: Goldenseal, orangeroot, yellowroot.

DESCRIPTION: Perennial.

>*Height:* To 15 inches.
>
>*Flowers:* A single, inconspicuous greenish white in spring, followed by red fruits; appears to perch between the leaves.
>
>*Leaves:* Wrinkled, palmate, resembling those of a maple.

HARVEST: Five-year-old roots.

CULTURE: Goldenseal thrives in deep, humus-rich, moist soil with good drainage. It is difficult to grow only in the wrong place. Where conditions are right, it spreads.

USE: It is an immune-system stimulant containing berberine.

COMMENTS: If used for more than two months, goldenseal may raise blood pressure. Pregnant women and those with high blood pressure should avoid this herb.

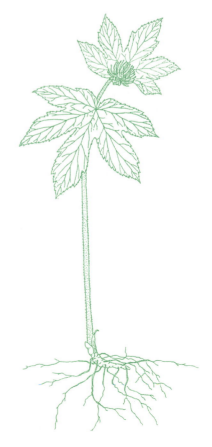

Goldenseal, sometimes called "the poor man's ginseng," has been collected so extensively and for so long that it is now near extinction in the wild. Its long tradition of treating mucous membrane infections and, more recently, myths about its ability to mask the presence of drugs in urine tests have extinguished what were once vast populations. It is now listed as endangered in six states.

Like ginseng, goldenseal is a rare woodland plant that ought to be grown in the home garden if for no other reason than to raise the number of its plants in the world. There are ethical sources (see Sources) that propagate this plant rather than collect it, as others do, from the wild— often in our national forests.

One spring I ordered some goldenseal rhizomes and then forgot all about doing so until the package arrived at the correct planting time, in fall. When I unwrapped them I understood the reason for the plant's common name: the young rhizomes were a bright golden yellow. The planting directions that came with them were specific. I followed them carefully, finding light shade with a deep layer of humus on moist but sloping ground. Spreading out the network of roots projecting from each rhizome, I made sure that the growth bud was about an inch below the soil surface.

It worked. Goldenseal's deeply crinkled, maple-shaped leaves now grow to about a foot tall. The leaves occur in twos. Between them, one small, greenish white spring flower, studded with yellow stamens, matures into a tight, bright scarlet berry cluster in fall. New plants formed along the outspread roots, and the goldenseal has grown into a handsome colony—too handsome for me to consider harvesting the five-year-old roots used in making medicine, except in direst need.

Nevertheless it is comforting to know that there is organically grown, fresh goldenseal available in the garden should such need arise. The anti-inflammatory properties of this bitter herb are many and well documented. For over a century, *The United States Pharmacopoeia* listed goldenseal as an astringent and antiseptic. Native Americans used goldenseal for a host of complaints. It was used as an eyewash, for skin wounds, for sore throats, for digestive complaints, and for recovery after childbirth. It is said to restore hormonal balance. Herbalists still use it externally to clean wounds and for eczema, ringworm, athlete's foot, itching, and conjunctivitis. Taken internally it is useful for colds, asthma, liver ailments, and digestive upsets. Goldenseal is considered a possible tumor-shrinker.

Today scientists regard goldenseal as an immune-system stimulant. They have identified berberine, an antibacterial and antifungal substance, as one of goldenseal's healing compounds. Berberine also occurs in the far more common and far easier to grow *Berberis vulgaris* and in *Mahonia* species. Apparently berberine kills bacteria that cause diarrhea, is effective against amoebic dysentery and giardiasis, and may even destroy cholera bacteria. Berberine also inhibits the growth of *Candida albicans*, the agent responsible for yeast infections. It does this by stimulating the white cells, or macrophages, the big white cells that engulf bacteria and viruses.

Gotu Kola

CENTELLA ASIATICA

BOTANICAL NAME: *Centella asiatica,* Apiaceae.

COMMON NAME: Gotu kola.

DESCRIPTION: Tender perennial.

>   *Height:* 3 to 4 inches.

>   *Flowers:* Tiny pink flowers are hidden by the leaves.

>   *Leaves:* Round on creeping stems.

HARVEST: All parts of the plant as needed.

CULTURE: Warm, rich, moist-to-wet soil.

USE: Gotu kola reduces inflammation and improves healing and immunity. It has been shown to reduce scarring when applied to inflamed wounds, and it has a positive effect on the circulatory system.

COMMENTS: It may cause skin irritation in some allergic individuals.

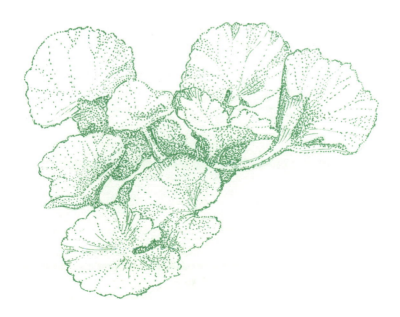

$\mathcal{A}$nything reputed to prevent aging and memory loss grabs my attention immediately. So when I saw plants of gotu kola for sale at the local garden center, I bought one and began reading everything I could to find out about it.

Gotu kola is highly regarded in Ayurvedic medicine. Fresh or dried leaves are used as a blood purifier to cure chronic skin conditions and to treat leprosy and nervous disorders. Its reputation as an antiaging herb stems from its positive effects on the circulatory system. It has been shown to reduce scarring.

One interesting culinary use of gotu kola is as a salad green. In Japan, its leaves are served raw in salads. This is triply appealing. First, eating gotu kola raw is the simplest and most direct way to take in all of its nutrients and beneficial compounds. Second, gotu kola thrives outside in hot weather. When lettuce turns bitter and bolts, gotu kola takes its place as an excellent source of salad greens. Third, it thrives on a windowsill over the winter.

Gotu kola is a pretty little creeping plant that forms new plants along its stems. It hails from tropical swampy areas around the world. In the garden it thrives in moist to wet semishade. Be sure to bring it in if you live in an area where the temperature drops to freezing. It makes a fine houseplant that you cannot possibly overwater.

Calm and Centered Tea

Green tea has more flavor than gotu kola. I made a mixture of these two tea leaves to get the flavor of green tea and the benefits of both.

1. Mix equal parts of dried gotu kola leaves and green tea leaves.
2. Put 2 teaspoons per 8 ounces of water into a pot; pour boiling water over.
3. Allow to steep 5 to 10 minutes.

Heartsease, Johnny-jump-up

VIOLA TRICOLOR

BOTANICAL NAME: *Viola tricolor,* Violaceae.

COMMON NAMES: Heartsease, Johnny-jump-up, wild pansy, love-in-idleness.

DESCRIPTION: Hardy annual.

Height: To 8 inches.

Flowers: Tricolor flowers are purple, lavender, and yellow. They, as well as the leaves, may be eaten.

Leaves: Scalloped, edible.

HARVEST: Freshly opened flowers on organically grown plants.

CULTURE: Plant in early spring for late-spring bloom; cut back when the temperature rises, for another flush of bloom in fall.

USE: It eases emotional pain. Serve the flowers in salads and fruit cups.

COMMENTS: Don't scoff until you've tried it.

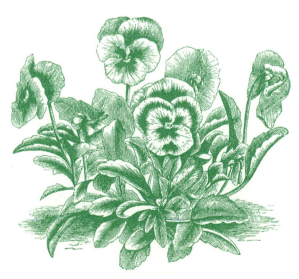

Yet mark'd I where the bolt of Cupid fell:
It fell upon a little western flower,
Before milk-white, now purple with love's wound,
And maidens call it love-in-idleness.
Fetch me that flower; the herb I shew'd thee once:
The juice of it on sleeping eye-lids laid
Will make or man or woman madly dote
Upon the next live creature that it sees.
   —Shakespeare, *A Midsummer-Night's Dream*

*T*he flowers that Shakespeare called love-in-idleness have more than one common name. Most often known as Johnny-jump-up, these flowers are also called heartsease—a reference to their role in folk medicine as a heart healer. Though I am convinced, for empirical reasons, that their reputation for healing emotional pain is deserved, I doubt I'll find scientific evidence to support this use.

There is plentiful evidence that pansies and violets are good for you in other ways. Their leaves and flowers are high in vitamins A and C. According to Dr. James Duke, pansies contain compounds that help in the treatment of glaucoma. And the German Commission E includes heartsease on its approved list as effective for mild seborrhoeic skin disorders when decoctions of the chopped herb are applied. Far more dramatically, *Viola tricolor* has been used by the Arabs as a remedy for scorpion stings for millennia.

So pansies and violets are not only safe to eat but healthful, and they are turning up in unexpected places—notably in the salads and sorbets served in trendy restaurants.

The sweetest perfume may belong to the sweet violet *(V. odorata)*, but my favorite member of the violet family is heartsease. Heartsease plants are freely available in garden centers both in spring and fall: just ask for Johnny-jump-ups. These hardy annuals thrive in cool weather. Planted in fall, they bloom again in spring.

To eat them or use them as edible garnish, make sure that they are free of pesticides. The best way to do this is to grow your own from seed (see Sources), rather than buy them. Then, make Heartsease Salad. Serve it to a brokenhearted friend and see for yourself if it doesn't help.

Heartsease Salad

Picking pretty heartsease flowers to fortify a garden salad seemed to me just the thing when I first served Hildegard von Bingen's Hyssop Chicken for Sadnesse (see page 126). If possible, wash the flowers and allow them to dry while they are still on the plant. To keep them absolutely fresh, pick just before serving.

½ cup lemon balm leaves
6–8 leaves of any garden lettuce
   Purslane, bee balm leaves, or gotu kola leaves, optional
6–8 heartsease flowers
   Thyme-Ginger Dressing (page 247)

1. Wash and spin-dry the leaves and lettuce; wash the heartsease flowers if they are not already clean. Wrap the greens and the flowers in linen towels, encase in a plastic bag, and crisp in the refrigerator.
2. Just before serving, toss the greens and arrange the flowers. Serve with Thyme-Ginger Dressing.

YIELD: 2 servings

Horehound,
White Horehound

MARRUBIUM VULGARE

BOTANICAL NAME: *Marrubium vulgare,* Lamiaceae.

COMMON NAMES: Horehound, white horehound.

DESCRIPTION: Perennial.

Height: To 30 inches.

Flowers: Small, off-white, with prominent stamens; they encircle the top stems in summer.

Leaves: Downy leaves are gray-green or white.

HARVEST: Leaves and flowers when the flowers bloom.

CULTURE: Zones 4 to 9. Needs perfect drainage, sun, protection from wind.

USE: For coughs and colds.

COMMENTS: While extremely large doses of horehound can cause heart irregularities, if you stick to three or four cups of tea or five or six doses of syrup, you'll be fine. Horehound is bitter.

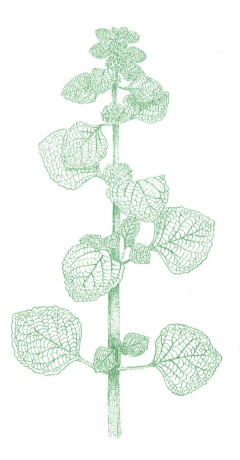

White horehound's use as an expectorant and cough medicine dates back to pharaonic times. Its efficacy as a remedy for coughs and colds has been documented over millennia—for example, in the writings of the Greek physician Galen and the medieval abbess Hildegard von Bingen.

Now modern research has found out why it works: a chemical in white horehound, marrubin, has phlegm-loosening properties. Used in Europe for decades, white horehound has been declared "an effective expectorant" by Varro E. Tyler, one of the country's foremost experts on plant drugs. The German Commission E includes horehound on its approved list for dyspeptic conditions and flatulence.

A good plant for pot culture, horehound is a perennial that grows best in full sun with some protection from wind in nearly neutral soil that is on the dry side. Although horehound is hardy in Zones 4 to 9, it is extremely sensitive to winter wetness. If you have heavy soil, amend it with chicken grit or grow horehound in a raised bed.

If you have plants that are established, wait until midspring when the weather is settled to divide them. Replant divisions one foot apart. When a plant begins vigorous growth, cut it back into a more compact shape. It will reach two feet.

If you can find it, silver horehound *(Marrubium incanum)*, hardy to Zone 6 with protection, is a beautiful ornamental. It has the same medicinal properties as its gray-green cousin.

Pick the leaves as needed.

Horehound Syrup

My efforts at making horehound candies failed. The candy never really got hard. That's when I decided to try making a syrup. This is simply a sugar syrup, flavored with horehound and spices. You may wish to experiment by adding other flavorings, such as cloves or lemon. This easy-to-make syrup can be combined with herbs in teas.

1 cup sugar
1 cup water
½ cup packed fresh horehound leaves

3 cardamom seeds, crushed
½-inch slice of fresh gingerroot, grated

1. Combine the sugar with the water in a saucepan; cook until the sugar is dissolved.
2. Add the horehound, cardamom seeds, and ginger.
3. Simmer 20 minutes. Strain through a fine filter.

NOTE: Add to echinacea tea for colds and coughs.

Hyssop

BOTANICAL NAME: *Hyssopus officinalis,* Lamiaceae.

COMMON NAME: Hyssop.

DESCRIPTION: Perennial.

> *Height:* To 2 inches.
>
> *Flowers:* Blue, white, or pink, in spikes.
>
> *Leaves:* Edible, small, dark green, narrow leaves are pointed.

HARVEST: Leaves as needed; for tea, cut the whole plant at flowering time.

CULTURE: Grow in full sun in light, well-drained, alkaline soil. Sow in spring and transplant seedling to 2 feet apart; divide in spring or start new plants from stem cuttings or wait until it self-sows. Hyssop can be grown indoors; to keep it trim and bushy, cut it back to around 8 inches after flowering. The plant is attractive to cabbage butterflies; grow near cabbage to lure them away from it.

USE: As a tea for upper respiratory ailments. Also, as an unusual flavoring.

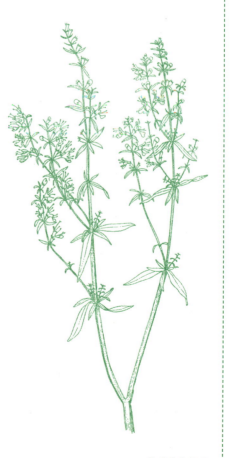

COMMENTS: Pregnant women should consult a doctor or herbalist before using the tea.

*P*retty hyssop's sternly flavored leaves appear throughout history as a remedy for upper respiratory ailments. Dioscorides prescribed hyssop in tea for coughs, wheezing, and shortness of breath. Hildegard von Bingen prescribed it as a lung cleanser used alone or combined with mullein to treat bronchitis.

Like horehound, hyssop contains constituents similar to camphor that make it useful as an expectorant and good for coughs. Modern investigation also suggests that hyssop inhibits the growth of the herpes simplex virus.

Despite its medicinal uses, hyssop is not the first herb you reach for in the kitchen. Its flavor is strong and dark—a bitter, peppery mint. After many frustrating attempts, I learned a bit about using it. Now I prefer it to sage for stuffing and find that it offsets the sweetness of fruit pies— especially peach. Try tossing a few leaves into cranberry sauce. In American Colonial times, the fresh leaves were used to flavor soups, stews, and stuffings and for tea.

In the formal garden, hyssop serves as a low hedge plant, attractive encircling other, taller herbs. In warm climates, it is evergreen. In colder places, it is up very early in spring. Keep it trim and bushy by cutting it back hard in midspring.

Hyssop Chicken for Sadnesse

Somewhere—I don't remember where—I read that Hildegard von Bingen, the twelfth-century German abbess, concocted a chicken dish with hyssop and wine to cure "sadnesse." Thus began a quest for a recipe I never found. I did learn a great deal about this tenth child, tithed to the church by her noble family. Lucky for her! Otherwise, she might have been so occupied with ten children of her own that she would never have written music or healed with herbs or theorized about man and God.

I thought that I could reconstruct her recipe using rather sweet white wines from the Bingen region, along with chicken and hyssop. After many truly colossal failures and a vast waste of wine and chicken (damn the hyssop), I hit upon a combination that might actually lift spirits. It did mine. Serve with Heartsease Salad (page 121).

   1 chicken (4–5 pounds)
   1 cup bread crumbs
  ½ cup chopped onion
   1 tablespoon chopped fresh hyssop
  ½ teaspoon (or slightly less) salt
     Plenty of pepper
   4 carrots, chopped
  ½ pound string beans, each snapped in two
 10 whole shallots, peeled (use the runts of your harvest)
   4 potatoes, peeled and cut in quarters
   1 cup strong chicken stock
   1 cup dry red wine
  ¼ cup cream, optional

1. Stuff the chicken with a dressing of the bread crumbs, onion, hyssop, and seasonings.
2. Place the chicken in the bottom of a Dutch oven or large covered pot. Cook, uncovered, in a 400° oven for 10 minutes. Turn down the heat to 325° and cook for 1 hour.
3. Remove the Dutch oven from the oven, lift the chicken out, and layer the vegetables in. Replace the chicken.
4. Pour in the chicken stock and wine.
5. Cook another 1½ hours.
6. Remove from the heat. Cool, then carve the chicken. Arrange the chicken and vegetables on a large platter.
7. Reduce the pan juices to a thin gravy. Adjust seasoning. Add the cream, if desired. Pass the gravy with the chicken and stuffing. Feel good.

YIELD: 6 servings

Hyssop-Peach Tart

Although my experiments with hyssop were mostly unsuccessful, this one hit the spot. The all-out sweetness of fresh peaches is made more interesting by a bit of hyssop sprinkled over the crust of this tart, which is nice with homemade peach ice cream.

FOR THE CRUST:

1½ cups flour

  6 teaspoons butter

 ¼ teaspoon salt

 ¼ cup sugar

    Up to ½ cup ice water

FOR THE FILLING:

  1 teaspoon very finely chopped hyssop

4–5 ripe peaches

2–3 tablespoons sugar

1. Preheat the oven to 350°.
2. With a pastry cutter, combine the flour, butter, salt, and sugar until the mixture clumps into pea-size pieces. Avoid overworking the dough and making it tough. Add just enough cold water so that you can make a ball of the dough. Place the dough in a bowl, cover it with a towel, and let it rest for 30 to 60 minutes in the refrigerator.
3. Roll the dough out and fit it into a 9- to 10-inch tart pan, spring-form pan, or cake pan.
4. Prebake it, using pie weights (or beans over parchment paper) for 15 minutes at 350°. Allow this crust to cool.
5. Sprinkle the hyssop over the bottom of the tart crust. Add peach slices in concentric rings, starting at the outside edge. Sprinkle liberally with sugar. Bake for 30 minutes.

YIELD: 4 to 6 servings

Lamb's-quarters

CHENOPODIUM ALBUM

BOTANICAL NAME: *Chenopodium album,* Chenopodaceae.

COMMON NAMES: Lamb's-quarters, lamb's lettuce.

DESCRIPTION: Annual.

Height: To 30 inches.

Flowers: Inconspicuous.

Leaves: Wedge-shaped leaves are edible.

HARVEST: In summer, as soon as there is enough to be worthwhile.

CULTURE: Easy in full sun and moist, fertile soil.

USE: Like spinach, but richer in vitamins A and C. It also contains calcium.

COMMENTS: As good as spinach and easier to grow.

OTHER SPECIES: Seeds are available for *Chenopodium giganteum,* a tall form of lamb's-quarters.

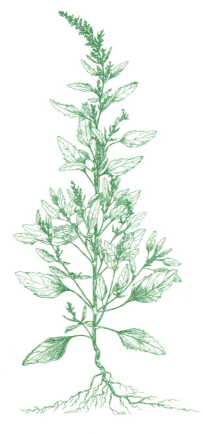

Years ago, I started a vast vegetable garden with the intention of becoming self-sufficient—immediately. In a single season, I learned to know intimately many of the diseases and insects that prey upon food crops. Carrots were misshapen, broccoli was wormy, and spinach was scarred by leaf miners.

I don't remember exactly when I

became aware of lamb's-quarters, but the notion of eating that particular wild green must have come from one of Bradford Angier's books. One day I looked up from my labors in the garden and there, like a lily in the field, was lamb's-quarters, abundant, perfect, and free for the picking.

It was, in my opinion, more delicious than spinach. Impervious to heat, it was far easier to grow. In fact, for many years I didn't plant it but cut it out of the fields and verges where it sprang up on its own.

Collecting seeds in late summer enables you to grow lamb's-quarters where you want it. Recently I found seeds of *Chenopodium giganteum* 'Magenta Spreen,' a tall, bicolored lamb's-quarters with a beautiful magenta blotch.

A rich source of vitamins A and C, as well as calcium, lamb's-quarters grows easily from seeds planted in spring. I wait until just after the last frost when the soil has warmed a bit to plant it.

Harvest leaves and young, tender stems as soon as they are big enough to be worth the effort. Cook lamb's-quarters exactly as you would spinach. Like spinach, great "messes" of lamb's-quarters shrink down to small masses of delicious greens.

Lamb's-quarters Crêpes

Every time I make crêpes, I remember this legend: the king of France, out hunting and hungry, came upon a poor shack in the woods and asked for food. The inhabitant, a young and beautiful maiden (of course), had little to offer—two eggs, some flour, and a bit of milk—but she was ingenious and combined them to make the first crêpes. As in the legend, this recipe takes very plain ingredients to produce a truly elegant dish. On a whim, I added lamb's-quarters leaves to the crêpe batter and found it turned out pretty, flecked green pancakes, complementing the white cheese sauce.

The spinach-Gruyère combination was inspired by a classic quiche. Why not go one step further and add some crumbled bacon over the sauce?

FOR THE CRÊPES:

2 cups flour

3 eggs

2 cups milk

3 tablespoons melted butter

Leaves from 4–5 sprigs of lamb's-quarters
2 tablespoons olive oil

FOR THE SAUCE:
 3 tablespoons butter
 3 tablespoons flour
1½ cups milk, heated almost to a boil
 1 cup Gruyère, grated

FOR THE LAMB'S-QUARTERS FILLING:
 2 tablespoons olive oil
½ cup shallots, cut fine
 4 cups chopped lamb's-quarters
 Salt and pepper

TO MAKE THE CRÊPES:

1. Sift the flour into a blender container, then add the other ingredients except the oil and blend until smooth. Refrigerate for 2 hours. Blend again.
2. Heat all the oil in a crêpe pan or small skillet until very hot. Pour a small amount of batter into the pan, tilt the pan so that the batter runs over the bottom to coat it evenly, and pour back the excess into the blender.
3. Cook 1 to 2 minutes on the first side, flip over and cook for 30 seconds, and remove the crêpe to a plate. Repeat until the batter is gone. Set aside.

TO MAKE THE SAUCE:

1. Melt the butter in a saucepan, stir in the flour, and combine with a wire whisk.
2. Slowly whisk in the hot milk until the mixture comes to a boil. Reduce the heat and stir in the grated cheese. Whisk until the sauce is smooth. Remove from heat.

TO FINISH:

1. Preheat the oven to 350°.
2. Heat the oil in a skillet. Add the shallots and cook for 3 to 5 minutes.

3. Add the lamb's-quarters. Cook until it is dark green and limp.
4. Mix the lamb's-quarters with ¾ cup of the cheese sauce. Season with salt and pepper to taste.
5. Place 2 tablespoons of the lamb's-quarters on each crêpe. Roll the crêpes one by one and place them on an ovenproof platter. When all the crêpes are gone or all lamb's-quarters have been used up, top with the cheese sauce and bake for about 25 minutes.

YIELD: 4 servings

Lamb's-quarters—Chickpea Curry

After spending a year in India, I found myself hopelessly addicted to spicy, Indian-style food. Both spinach and chickpeas are classic ingredients in Indian cuisine. Purists may argue that my version isn't the genuine article, but having frozen Curry in a Hurry on hand makes this ersatz curry spicy enough to satisfy my needs. Serve this "curry" over rice or as a side dish.

1 tablespoon olive oil
2 tablespoons Curry in a Hurry (page 58)
1 tablespoon curry powder
1 pound (4 cups) lamb's-quarters, chopped, washed, and drained
Salt and pepper
3 cups cooked, shelled chickpeas, or 2 cans, rinsed and drained but not dried

1. Heat the oil in a 3-quart saucepan. Add the Curry in a Hurry. Cook 3 minutes.
2. Add the curry powder. Cook until brown—not more than a minute.
3. Add the lamb's-quarters. Season with salt and pepper.
4. Cook until the lamb's-quarters are dark and tender, 5 to 10 minutes.
5. Add the chickpeas and heat through. Adjust the seasoning and serve.

NOTE: Serve with Joan's Mast-O-Khiar (page 208).

YIELD: 4 to 6 servings

Lavender

LAVANDULA ANGUSTIFOLIA SYN. *LAVANDULA OFFICINALIS*

BOTANICAL NAME: *Lavandula angustifolia,* Lamiaceae.

COMMON NAMES: Lavender, English or common lavender.

DESCRIPTION: Evergreen (gray) shrub.

Height: To 2 feet.

Flowers: Lavender blue in summer.

Leaves: Aromatic, narrow, gray.

HARVEST: The flowers before they open, in the tight bud stage.

CULTURE: Zones 5 to 10 in neutral, well-drained soil with average moisture.

USE: Sedative, sachet.

COMMENTS: A good container or over-a-wall plant.

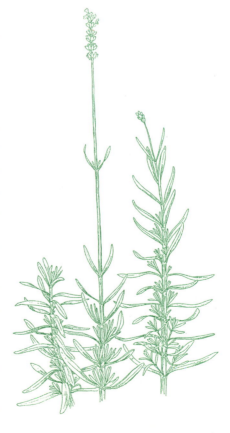

*I*t's official. The German Commission E says it is so: lavender flowers are on its approved list as effective for treating insomnia, mood disturbances, restlessness, and nervous stomach.

Apparently lavender's highly aromatic oil, long used to scent perfumes and soaps, helps to slow down nerve impulses. Phytochemical expert Dr. James Duke, author of *The Green Pharmacy,* writes that the components in lavender oil interrupt the interaction of cells with each other, thus helping to reduce irritability and bring on sleep. Christine Malcolm, executive director of the Aroma Research Institute of America, states: "Olfactory stimulation has the capacity to produce an immediate effect on the nervous system." In other words, when inhaled, lavender's lovely scent and its capacity to slow down nerve impulses go right to the brain.

While highly concentrated lavender oil is toxic if ingested, there are a number of very pleasant ways to benefit from lavender's aroma. Set out a potpourri of lavender and other aromatics. Put sachets of lavender in your drawers or tumble them with clothes in the dryer. Lavender oil (in small quantities) can be absorbed through the skin. Use lavender oil or muslin bags of lavender buds to scent bathwater. Or make refreshing Lavender Spritzer (page 137) to use on your skin.

Because lavender is very slow to grow from seed, buy a plant. Place it in full sun and rapidly draining, neutral soil. Acid soil needs liming to support lavender.

To sweeten my acid soil, I have put to good use chips of cement that crumble out of a path. On the advice of herb expert Holly Shimizu, I have also added bags of chicken grit to lighten the clay soil. The best advice for maintaining a healthy lavender plant came from James Adams, curator of the National Herb Garden at the U.S. National Arboretum. He recommends mulching around lavender plants with a light-reflecting layer of gravel or chicken grit.

It is not surprising that lavender, thriving as it does with fast drainage and in light, dry soil, also grows well in containers. *Lavandula* 'Compacta Nana,' a dwarf form, is a good type for this use.

While lavender *(Lavandula angustifolia)* is hardy in Zones 5 to 10, it suffers in very hot and humid places such as the Gulf Coast and may need replacing annually. If that is the case, try the cultivar 'Lady' that has been bred for use as an annual. Mulching with gravel or light-colored stones that reflect light helps. My favorite lavender is *Lavandula intermedia* 'Grosso,' for its very long flower spikes and sturdiness in my Zone 7 garden. If the flowers are cut, it reblooms.

Some species of lavender are very tender. French lavender *(Lavandula stoechas)*, said to have a stimulating effect similar to that of rosemary, is hardy only in Zone 8 and up. Fringed lavender *(Lavandula dentata)* is hardy only in Zones 9 and 10. Elsewhere, these plants have to be brought in over winter.

New lavender cultivars are constantly being bred. One repeat-bloomer is *Lavender angustifolia* 'Sharon Roberts.'

To harvest lavender, cut stems before the flowers open, when the buds are in tight rows. Hang the stems upside down to dry. Then you can either strip the highly aromatic buds from the stems for use in potpourri or sachets or in the seasoning mix Herbes de Provence (page 93).

Lavender Ice Cream

Experimenting with making lavender-flavored crème brûlée led to this simple and delicious ice cream. It is absolutely delicious.

4 egg yolks
½ cup sugar
1 teaspoon cornstarch
2 cups half-and-half
1 heaping teaspoon fresh, chopped lavender leaves

1. Combine the egg yolks, sugar, and cornstarch in a mixing bowl. Use a mixer to beat until the mixture is nearly white. Set aside.
2. Combine the half-and-half and the lavender leaves in a pan and heat almost to boiling.
3. With the mixer running (or while stirring), ladle some of the hot cream into the egg yolk mixture. Slowly add the rest.
4. Return this mixture to the pan and heat until it thickens. *Do not boil!*
5. Strain and chill the mixture.
6. When the mixture is cold, pour it into an ice-cream maker and process.

YIELD: 6 servings

> **TIP**
>
> *James Adams uses lavender as a strewing herb—in his car. In summer, when a car heats up inside, the lavender gives off a delightful aroma that is soothing after a hard day's work. (Adams says that when he has pressing brainwork to do, he strews with rosemary.)*

Lavender Crème Brûlée

Stephen Sands, by day a nuclear physicist, leads a double life. When night falls, he dons a toque and turns into a chef. He demonstrated the preparation of this lavender crème brûlée in one of his classes at l'Academie de Cuisine. The addition of lavender leaves—not flowers—adds, in his words, "another dimension of subtle flavor and helps offset the richness of the dessert." If you are organized enough to think a week in advance, you can make Lavender Sugar (page 137) for the caramelized topping. Chefs often use small blowtorches for the caramelizing process, but a friend who lives in Catalan country, where crème brûlée originated and is called "crème catalan," gave me a salamander, a kind of branding iron, and I've found that it works beautifully. Preparation also requires six-ounce ramekins.

1 quart heavy cream
½ vanilla bean, or 2 teaspoons vanilla extract
3–4 large sprigs of lavender
½ cup sugar plus additional for the topping, or use Lavender
   Sugar (recipe follows) for the topping
10 egg yolks (save the whites for other uses)
   Pinch of salt

1. Preheat the oven to 325°. Pour the cream into a medium saucepan. Split the vanilla bean in half and scrape the seeds of the bean into the cream. (If you are using vanilla extract instead, you will add it later.) Add the sprigs of lavender and scald the cream over medium heat until you see small bubbles on the sides of the pan.

2. Meanwhile, in a medium-size bowl, whisk the sugar into the egg yolks until the mixture is pale yellow. Once the cream has reached the scalding point, remove from the heat and strain out the lavender sprigs. Slowly temper the hot cream into the egg mixture. Stir in the salt (and the vanilla extract, if using in place of vanilla seeds).

3. Heat 1 quart of water to boiling.

4. Line a baking sheet (or baking dish) with several layers of paper towel. Arrange eight 6-ounce ramekins on the pan and pour the mixture into the ramekins. Pour hot water into the pan until it comes halfway up the sides of the ramekins. Cover the pan with foil. Bake

until just set, 30 to 50 minutes. Start checking early; baking time depends on the thickness and depth of the ramekins and baking pan.

5. Carefully remove the pan from the oven; let the ramekins cool in the water bath. Remove, cover with plastic, and refrigerate 2 hours or up to 2 days.

6. When ready to serve, ignite a blowtorch, sprinkle a thin, even layer of sugar over the custards, and with a slow sweeping motion guide the flame directly on the surface of the first custard. The nozzle should be 3 to 4 inches from the surface, with the tip of the flame licking the sugar. The sugar will melt slowly at first and then caramelize. As soon as the entire surface is glossy brown, move to the next custard.

YIELD: 8 servings

Lavender Sugar

It takes a few days to coax the lavender scent into the sugar. This can be used for the caramelized topping of Lavender Crème Brûlée (see recipe above).

    15–20 young, *dry* lavender leaves
        1 cup sugar

1. Place the lavender leaves in a covered container (a recycled cottage cheese container is perfect).
2. Cover with the sugar. Tamp the leaves with a wooden spoon.
3. Cover the container and shake once a day for several days.

Lavender Spritzer

Using the procedure for sun tea, I made this spritzer to use on the skin anytime. It is especially refreshing after a shower in summer.

1. Mix 1 tablespoon dried lavender buds with 2 cups water in a glass jar.
2. Set in the sun for one day to steep.
3. Transfer to a spray bottle. Keep it in the fridge.

Lemon Balm

BOTANICAL NAME: *Melissa officinalis,* Lamiaceae.

COMMON NAME: Lemon balm.

DESCRIPTION: Perennial that is semievergreen in warm winters.

    Height: To 2 feet.

    Flowers: Small, inconspicuous white.

    Leaves: Edible, nearly heart-shaped, scalloped.

HARVEST: If drying for tea, cut before flowers form on a dry, sunny day in summer; dry in airy shade as quickly as possible. Cut the stems to the ground; lemon balm will resprout and probably yield a second or third harvest.

CULTURE: Zones 4 to 9, sun or light shade in average soil.

USE: Contains compounds that alleviate headache, depression, anxiety. Use for salads, desserts, teas.

COMMENTS: If you can't grow this one, turn in your trowel.

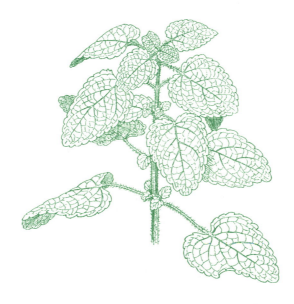

One of the most useful herbs in the garden because it tastes wonderful and has great healing properties, lemon balm is also one of the easiest to grow. Once you have it, it will pop up around the garden with a persistence that might be annoying were lemon balm not so wonderfully useful.

Compounds in lemon balm's leaves calm anxiety, lift depression, and are thought to prevent migraine. The German Commission E includes it on its approved list for nervous sleeping disorders. One form of lemon balm with a very high content of essential oils and a bushy habit can be grown from seed (see Sources). It is called 'Quedlinburger Niederliegende.'

Start seeds six weeks before the last frost in your area and transplant the seedlings out after all danger of frost has passed. By midsummer, you can begin harvesting leaves for salads, fruit salads, vegetables, sangria, and to use in dressings (see the recipe for Lemon Balm Dressing). By fall, you should be able to harvest enough leaves to dry for use with other herbs in tea mixtures. The dried leaves keep their aroma but lose their flavor. They add a pleasant lemony aroma to potpourri.

Lemon balm is a perennial that grows to just under two feet tall. I grow it in part shade, and I suspect that the farther south lemon balm grows, the more shade it tolerates. As long as it has decent drainage, it is not fussy about soil and hardy in Zones 4 to 9. In its second year in the garden and thereafter it produces small, insignificant white flowers, after which seeds form, ensuring you lifelong lemon balm. Thus, when older plants get too woody and die, very likely you will be able to find replacements already growing in the garden.

Lemon balm's vigor and easy-growing temperament make it useful in containers and window boxes. I haven't tried overwintering it indoors, but I think it would do just fine.

Bread Salad with Garden Thinnings

Like stone soup, bread salad is a deliciously satisfying way to make use of whatever the garden produces. There is no hard-and-fast recipe. For me, it's a late-summer ritual meal from the thinnings of fall salad greens—mizuma, Italian dandelion, spinach, and lettuces. At that time of year I always find some basil and Italian parsley and lots of little cherry tomatoes that have self-sown their way around the garden. I have made it with a lovely, crusty rosemary-olive bread, but almost any good-quality home-style bread that is a day old works fine.

FOR THE LEMON BALM VINAIGRETTE (ABOUT ¾ CUP):
½ cup extra virgin olive oil
3½ tablespoons lemon juice
1 teaspoon salt
20 lemon balm leaves

FOR THE SALAD:
4 cups day-old bread, cut into 1-inch cubes
1 red onion, chopped
2 cups halved cherry tomatoes
2 cups salad garden thinnings, washed and with the roots removed
3 tablespoons of any combination of chopped basil, Italian parsley, and perilla

1. Blend all the ingredients for the dressing into a beautiful, pale green emulsion. Set aside.
2. In a large bowl, toss the bread cubes with ½ cup of the vinaigrette. Let the bread stand for a half hour to soak up the dressing.
3. Add the onion, tomatoes, salad garden thinnings, chopped herbs, and, finally, the remaining dressing. Toss gently and serve immediately.

YIELD: 2 servings

Lemon Balm Dressing

The addition of almost any herb to vinaigrette creates a more interesting dressing. I think this one is excellent for early spring salads. It is also a terrific marinade. Try it for marinating briefly blanched broccoli florets.

½ cup olive oil
¼ cup freshly squeezed lemon juice

2 tablespoons chopped fresh lemon balm leaves (6–10)
¼ teaspoon Dijon mustard
1 teaspoon salt, or to taste

Place all the ingredients in a blender and blend until the dressing is a smooth yellow-green.

YIELD: ¾ cup dressing

Lemongrass

CYMBOPOGON CITRATUS

BOTANICAL NAME: *Cymbopogon citratus,* Poaceae.

COMMON NAME: Lemongrass.

DESCRIPTION: Tender perennial.

Height: To 4 feet.

Flowers: Doesn't flower in cultivation.

Leaves: Long, gray-green blade arises from a bulbous culm at the base.

HARVEST: As needed or in fall when the grass is taken indoors for the winter.

CULTURE: Zones 8 to 10; sun, average soil and moisture.

USE: As an antifungal and for a headache tea. Also for flavoring.

COMMENTS: A very ornamental grass; grows rapidly in hot weather.

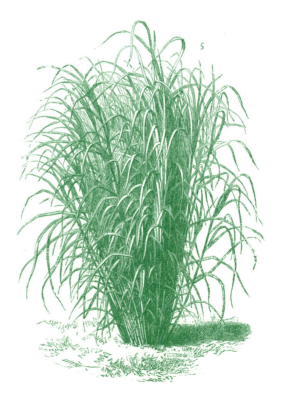

Lemongrass, a handsome ornamental grass that grows to over three feet tall, is a graceful backdrop in an herb garden. During the growing season, all you have to do to have lemongrass for cooking is twist off a stalk from the base of the plant.

Lemongrass shares the gray-green foliage color of lavender, but not lavender's hardiness. After frost, it turns a beautiful amber color and makes a superb winter accent, but, in my Zone 7 garden, it never wakes up again in the spring. To survive, it has to be dug up every year in mid-October, about the time of our first air frost. I've tried overwintering it in a cold frame, with no luck.

Those with room enough in a sunny window for a big pot can dig up the whole grass and bring it inside for the winter. In my house, there's room only for a division. I lift the whole grass in fall and divide it, using a pruning saw to get through the roots. One rooted portion will spend the winter in a pot on my windowsill. This will be transplanted back into a sunny spot in the garden next spring, after all danger of frost has passed. By fall, it will have grown large again and the process will be repeated.

The rest gets harvested. The part of the grass used in cooking is the base of the culm—the bottom nine inches or so of each blade. If you trim off the grassy tops and the roots, you will end up with what they sell in the supermarket, something that looks like a very stiff, plump green onion.

Lemongrass is a lusty grower. You will have so many of these stiff culms that storage becomes an issue. For more immediate use, within a month or two of harvest, you can stand several of these in a glass with an inch of water on the kitchen counter. They not only keep well, they often root. Chop up the rest. The classic method is to whack the culm with the broad side of a big knife to tenderize it and then chop it into fine shreds. If you are planning to eat the lemongrass rather than use it to flavor food, remove the tough outer leaves. This is always upsetting because the tender center is so very much smaller than what you started with. You will probably feel like you are throwing most of the grass away. You are, but if you grow your own, there is plenty more.

Freeze or dry chopped lemongrass. Frozen lemongrass keeps for about six months. Use the dried lemongrass within one year. Add some to potpourri.

I used to think that only the base of the grass was useful, and I would cut off the long grass blades and compost them. Then Lydia Fontenot, a grower and crafter of herbs in Louisiana (where lemongrass is hardy), taught me how to make use of the whole grass. Now I braid the blades or tie them into knots to be snipped off into teas, steamed with vegetables, or tucked into a roasting chicken for a subtle lemony flavor. Tied with a ribbon, a braid or a bowlful of knots makes a nice gift.

Lemongrass contains citral, a compound that fights fungal infections such as athlete's foot. Drink several cups of lemongrass tea every day and save the leaves or tea bags to apply to the infection.

In experiments with rats given a chemical known to cause colon cancer, scientists have found that lemongrass inhibits the number of abnormal cells likely to grow into cancerous tumors.

Lemongrass Braid for Tea

1. Take a sheaf of fresh lemongrass blades and fasten them at one end.
2. Separate the sheaf into three sections and braid them together.
3. Tie with a blade of lemongrass.

NOTE: To make the tea, snip off an inch or two of the braid as needed—about 1 tablespoon per cup. Steep for 5 to 10 minutes. Serve with honey and a lemon wedge.

Lemongrass Soup Asia Nora

Nora Pouillon's restaurants, Nora and Asia Nora, are noted for haute cuisine using only the freshest organic ingredients in season. This delicate clear soup is light and lovely all by itself, or you can pass around rice or noodles to spoon into it. Better yet, spoon stir-fried vegetables, chicken, or shrimp into bowls and pour this broth over them.

2 tablespoons olive oil
8 ounces (or more) shrimp shells
1 tablespoon chopped green onion
2 teaspoons finely chopped garlic

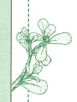

LEMONGRASS BOWS

1. Take a fresh, long lemongrass blade and wrap it around three fingers.
2. Use the last 10 inches to tie the bow.
3. Stack the bows in a collander in a warm, airy place until they dry.

NOTE: To use, tuck several into a roasting chicken for a lemony-chicken flavor. Or add 1 to 3 bows to the water in which broccoli is to be cooked or blanched. Not only does the broccoli taste better, the kitchen smells better.

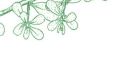

 1 tablespoon finely chopped ginger
 2 quarts chicken stock
 3 stems lemongrass, smashed
   Lime juice (be careful not to add too much)
1½ tablespoons nuoc mam (Vietnamese fish sauce)
 ½ teaspoon coriander seeds
 1 whole red chili
 4 sprigs cilantro
 1 lime leaf, optional
 1 tablespoon minced Thai basil or mint, optional
   Salt
   Brown sugar

1. Heat the oil and sauté shrimp shells until they turn red-pink.
2. Add the onion, garlic, and ginger and sauté briefly.
3. Add the chicken stock, lemongrass, nuoc nam, lime juice, coriander seeds, and chili and bring to a simmer.
4. Add the cilantro, lime leaf, and Thai basil or mint.
5. Simmer gently for 15 to 20 minutes.

6. Adjust the seasoning with salt, additional lime juice, and a pinch of brown sugar. Strain.

YIELD: 6 to 8 servings

Romy's Tom Khar

Yale law student Romy Mancini shared the recipe for this wonderful Thai soup. Rice is served as an accompaniment, creating a hearty main course. Once, at the last minute, I decided to serve the soup over rice as a sauce. After everything had cooked, I strained out the shrimp and vegetables and reduced the broth by boiling it until it thickened. This recipe works both ways.

2 cups chicken broth
1 packet Taste of Thai Coconut Ginger soup mix (there are two packets in each package)
1 chili pepper, chopped fine, or 1 teaspoon dried red pepper
1 bunch cilantro
2–3 stalks lemongrass, the outer layers peeled away and the tender inside cut into long, fine threads
2 cans unsweetened light coconut milk (*not* sweetened coconut milk)
Chicken breast (½–1 pound), cut into bite-size pieces
1 red sweet pepper, diced
½ pound mushrooms
¼ cup lime juice
4 cups cooked rice or noodles

1. In a 3-quart saucepan, boil the broth with the soup mix.
2. Add the chili pepper, the stems of the cilantro cut into tiny pieces (reserve the leaves), and the lemongrass. Then add the coconut milk. Bring to a boil.
3. Add the chicken. When it is halfway done, after 4 minutes, add the red sweet pepper.
4. After two or three minutes, add the mushrooms and lime juice.

5. Before serving the soup, sprinkle the reserved cilantro leaves over it.

6. Pass around a bowl of rice (or noodles) to spoon into the soup.

NOTE: You can also remove the chicken and vegetables while the broth reduces, and then return them to the broth and serve over rice.

YIELD: 4 servings

Red Snapper Fillet with Lemongrass

Jim Adams of the National Arboretum is a renowned host and cook. He suggests this dish for a pleasant dinner for two.

¼–½ pound fillet of red snapper
     Olive oil
     1-inch piece of gingerroot, peeled and sliced thin
1 stalk lemongrass, sliced in half lengthwise

1. Lay the fish skin side down in a lightly oiled pan.

2. Lay the circles of ginger in a row down the center of the fish.

3. Place ½ of the lemongrass, cut side down, on either side of the ginger.

4. Cover the pan tightly with aluminum foil. Bake for 15 to 20 minutes, or until fish flakes with a fork, in a 325° oven.

YIELD: 2 servings

Lemon Verbena

ALOYSIA TRIPHYLLA SYN. LIPPIA CITRIODORA

BOTANICAL NAME: *Aloysia triphylla* syn. *Lippia citriodora,* Verbenaceae.

COMMON NAME: Lemon verbena.

DESCRIPTION: Tender shrub.

> *Height:* To 6 feet.
>
> *Flowers:* Small, in white clusters at branch tips.
>
> *Leaves:* Long, narrow, gray-green. They are lemon-scented and edible.

HARVEST: As needed; for tea, cut a stem and brew with the leaves.

CULTURE: Zone 9 to 10, moderately rich soil with excellent drainage.

USE: For a sedative tea that helps headaches; for flavoring.

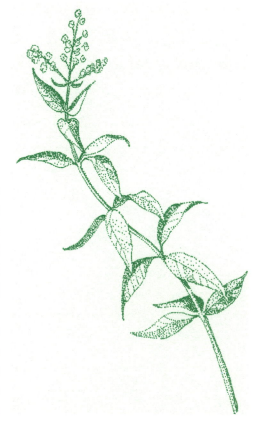

*E*llen O'Hara (Scarlett's mother) wore clothing that always exhaled a faint breath of lemon verbena. Dried lemon verbena leaves hold their perfume for years and scent linens and clothing delightfully. Not gardening in Tara's warm climate, where this South American plant is hardy in the ground, I've never had copious harvests.

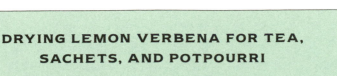
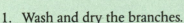

**DRYING LEMON VERBENA FOR TEA,
SACHETS, AND POTPOURRI**

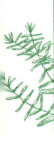

1. Wash and dry the branches.
2. Remove the leaves from the stems.
3. Lay the leaves out on a cookie sheet and place in a 200° oven for 5 minutes (or 2 to 3 minutes longer, until dry).

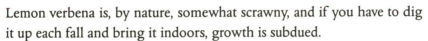

Lemon verbena is, by nature, somewhat scrawny, and if you have to dig it up each fall and bring it indoors, growth is subdued.

Two plants supply enough for culinary use, with a few leaves left over for potpourri or sachets. I've chopped up a leaf or two and tossed them into fruit salad or mixed them with fruit in yogurt smoothies. I've poured boiling water over fresh or dry leaves for a mildly sedating tea. I've even tossed a few leaves into bathwater. By far my favorite use for these aromatic leaves is in a lovely, lemony crème brûlée.

Lemon verbena is hardy only to Zone 9—or a climate with winters that don't get colder than 25 degrees Fahrenheit. You might be able, with luck and mulch, to squeak it through a Zone 8 winter, but it will certainly drop its leaves when the weather gets cold.

Where it can stay in the ground, lemon verbena will reach a rather leggy six feet or more. Where winters are colder, the plants have to be potted up each fall before the first frost and brought inside into a sunny window. This tends to keep the plant at about three feet, but puts it close at hand for winter cooking.

I have never seen seeds for lemon verbena offered. To get started with lemon verbena, buy a plant. If you plan to grow it in a container, mix sand or perlite into rich soil for good drainage and place it in a sunny place. Or place lemon verbena in the ground in a sunny, well-drained site. I've never done it, but they say lemon verbena starts easily from root cuttings taken in spring.

Mellow Yellow Crème Brûlée

Trying to intensify both the lemon flavor and the mood-enhancing effect of this crème brûlée, I added two herbs—lemon balm for its antidepressant, antioxidant properties, and lemon verbena, for its calming properties. The result was a lovely, delicate crème with a mellower taste than that of real lemon. The custard will keep in the fridge for two days, but the caramelized topping will stay crisp for only two hours or so in dry conditions. For extra flavor, make Lemon Verbena Sugar (recipe follows) for the topping.

½ cup sugar, plus ¾ cup additional for the caramelized topping (or use Lemon Verbena Sugar [recipe follows] for the topping)
3 eggs plus 3 yolks
2½ cups milk or half-and-half or cream
1 vanilla bean, seeds removed, or 1 teaspoon vanilla extract
2 tablespoons chopped fresh lemon verbena
6–8 fresh leaves lemon balm, chopped

1. Preheat the oven to 300°. Select an ovenproof pan large enough to hold 8 ramekins or a custard dish. Heat water in a kettle to boiling.
2. Beat the sugar and the eggs until the mixture is a soft yellow. Set aside.
3. Heat the milk with the vanilla, lemon verbena, and lemon balm until this mixture is almost boiling.
4. Stirring constantly, slowly pour some of the hot milk mixture into the sugar mixture. Return the sugar mixture to the pan and cook on low heat until it has thickened.
5. Pour the custard through a chinoise or fine mesh strainer. Then divide it among the ramekins.
6. Place the ramekins on the pan in the oven and pour boiling water into the pan to make a water bath halfway up the sides. Bake 20 to 25 minutes, until the custard is set but still jiggly in the center.
7. Chill the custard at least 3 hours.
8. Top the custard with the sugar and place under the broiler (or use a salamander or torch) until caramelized—about 5 minutes.

YIELD: 8 servings

Lemon Verbena Sugar

   1 cup sugar
5–6 dry lemon verbena leaves

1. Combine the sugar and the leaves in a container (a recycled yogurt or cottage cheese container works fine) and shake well.
2. Shake daily for 4 to 5 days. Use to top crème brûlée, in icings, or in teas.

Lovage

LEVISTICUM OFFICINALE

BOTANICAL NAME: *Levisticum officinale,* Apiaceae.

COMMON NAME: Lovage.

DESCRIPTION: Perennial.

    Height: 3 to 4 feet.

    Flowers: Small, yellow umbels produce edible, medicinal seeds.

    Leaves: Edible, pungent, celery-green leaves and stalks.

HARVEST: Leaves at any time; seeds when ripe; 2- to 3-year-old roots just before the flowers open.

CULTURE: Zones 4 to 8; sun to part shade; rich, moist, well-drained soil.

USE: Cystitis tea, flatulence remedy, indigestion remedy. A handy and uncommon vegetable.

COMMENTS: Do not use medicinally if you are pregnant or suffering from kidney disease.

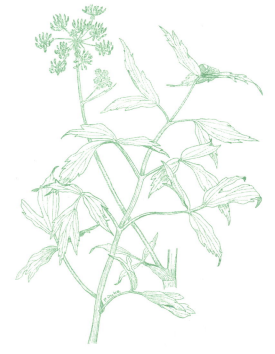

*L*ovage resembles a giant celery that has funneled all of its energy into making leaves instead of stalks. Celery green, the leaves and stalks are pretty enough to earn a place in the flower garden. Just be sure to site lovage behind shorter plants; it will reach three to six feet, depending upon the richness of the soil.

Lovage has a bigger-than-celery taste, too. Its pungent leaves deepen the flavor of soups and stews. The purple tips of young growth are especially appealing in spring salads, and all season long, fresh leaves serve as a ready source of salad greens. The summer flowers are a lovely, edible garnish. A salt substitute, dried leaves season fish; they are a pleasant alternative to dill.

Serve the stems as an uncommon vegetable. Simply steam and season with butter, salt, and pepper. Just as you would with celery, chop stems and toss them into stews and soups. Or skewer them for vegetable kebabs. They can also be candied.

In addition to leaves and stems, lovage produces small, yellow edible flowers, followed by tasty seeds. Sprinkle the seeds over mashed potatoes or bake them in or on bread or crackers.

Lovage seeds and roots, used since ancient times as digestives, are the parts of this plant considered medicinally efficacious. The German Commission E includes lovage root on its approved list as an irrigation therapy for lower urinary tract infections. Some herbalists formulate decoctions of these parts to treat cystitis and kidney stones.

While lovage is far easier to grow than celery, it doesn't care for hot, dry sites or excessive heat. Give it the best soil you have and a little shade if your garden gets a hot-climate summer. I suspect that lovage does not survive long in the deep South.

Lovage and Tomatoes

Juicy tomatoes complement lovage's strong personality—and vice versa. Marinate fresh-from-the-garden tomatoes in lovage-flavored vinaigrette. It is a refreshing departure from the classic summer combo of basil and tomatoes.

¼ cup olive oil

1½ tablespoons lemon juice

Pinch of dried mustard

Salt and pepper

¼ cup finely chopped lovage leaves

4 garden tomatoes, sliced, or 8 to 10 cherry tomatoes

1. Combine the oil, lemon juice, and mustard.
2. Add salt and pepper to taste.
3. Mix in the lovage leaves.
4. Pour the dressing over sliced or cherry tomatoes and allow to marinate at least 1 hour.

YIELD: 4 servings

Cold Lovage-Potato Soup

A little lovage goes a long way. I learned this the hard way after Washington chef Nora Pouillon suggested the combination and I labored to find the right blend. The amount in this great summer soup is just right. The lovage asserts itself, but graciously; it doesn't overwhelm.

1 teaspoon butter

½ cup onion, chopped

½ cup lovage, chopped leaves and stalk (about 3 stalks)

2 carrots, chopped

2 potatoes, cut into quarters

1 small zucchini, peeled and cut into chunks

1 bay leaf

3 cups chicken stock

Salt and pepper

1 cup half-and-half, optional

1. Melt the butter in a saucepan and add the onion. Cook gently about 5 minutes until the onion is soft. Add the lovage. Cook 5 minutes.
2. Add the carrots and cook 5 minutes. Add the potatoes, zucchini,

bay leaf, and chicken stock. Cook about 30 minutes, or until all of the vegetables are soft enough to blend. Season with salt and pepper. Cool.

3. In a blender, whir the soup until it is creamy. Adjust the seasoning. Chill.

4. If desired, add the half-and-half before serving (this will bring the yield to 5 servings).

YIELD: 4 or 5 servings

TIPS

- *Rub lovage leaf around the salad bowl.*
- *Use the hollow young stems of lovage for straws when serving Bloody Marys.*
- *Crumble dried lovage leaves (mixed with dried parsley) over vegetables as a salt substitute.*

Mexican Mint,
Mexican Marigold

BOTANICAL NAME: *Tagetes lucida,* Asteraceae.

COMMON NAMES: Mexican mint, Mexican marigold, Mexican tarragon.

DESCRIPTION: A tender perennial.

>*Height:* To 15 inches.

>*Flowers:* Yellow, in late summer.

>*Leaves:* Narrow, glossy.

HARVEST: Take clippings as needed.

CULTURE: Zones 8 and higher. Grow in full sun, in ordinary soil with good drainage.

USE: A tarragon substitute.

COMMENTS: Very tolerant of heat and humidity.

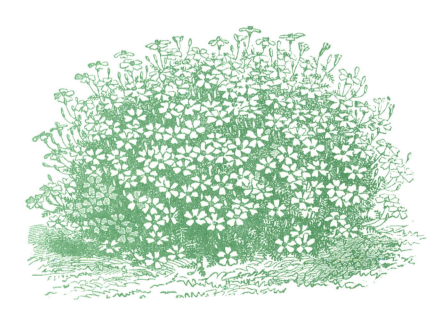

$\mathcal{B}$efore I found Mexican mint, many a tarragon expired in my garden—moping through a season or two, if that, and then disappearing between winter and spring. Southern Perennials & Herbs, a nursery in Mississippi that specializes in plants that tolerate heat, recommended Mexican mint as a tarragon substitute in places where tarragon doesn't thrive. I bought three. One went out into the garden to see if it would survive the winter. Another went into the cold frame and the third was a houseplant in a west window. The outside plants died in what was a mild winter in Zone 7. The houseplant died, too, but that was my fault, because I inadvertently allowed it to dry out.

In addition to anise-scented leaves that substitute admirably for tarragon, Mexican mint produces golden yellow, single marigold flowers that are as lovely as garnishes, or tossed into salads, as they are in the garden.

Site Mexican mint in sun, in well-drained soil. It forms an airy cushion of long, aromatic leaves studded with golden flowers. It also makes a fine subject for a container.

To harvest leaves for drying, cut back in early summer when the plant is in active growth. The small leaves dry quickly. When they are thoroughly dry, place them in an airtight bottle and keep it out of the light until you are ready to use the herb.

Mexican Mint and Watercress Butter

I've tried just about every herb in a butter, but this one is special. You can mix this delicious butter with a mortar and pestle, but a food processor or blender works fine, too. For a fancy garnish, push this butter through a pastry bag, making flowery medallions. Chill or freeze these until ready to serve with filet mignon or to float on soup.

    6 tablespoons butter (cool)
1½ tablespoons chopped Mexican mint
    1 tablespoon chopped watercress
    1 tablespoon lemon juice
      Salt and pepper

1. Pound the butter in the mortar until it is smooth.
2. Add the Mexican mint and watercress and pound until smooth.
3. Work in the lemon juice.
4. Add salt and pepper to taste.

Mexican Mint Hollandaise

This recipe is perfect with beautiful grass-green asparagus. It puts them over the top. Purists may balk at the microwave step, but I find that it thickens recalcitrant sauces and cooks the egg into the bargain. Tarragon may be substituted for the Mexican mint. This recipe makes about ¼ cup of sauce—enough for 2. You can double the recipe.

> 1 egg yolk (3 for a double recipe)
> Pinch of salt
> 1 teaspoon lemon juice
> 1 tablespoon chopped Mexican mint
> ¼ cup butter

1. Put the egg yolk, salt, and lemon juice in the blender and blend for a few seconds.
2. Add the Mexican mint to the melted butter.
3. While the blender is on, add the mint mixture in a thin stream. If the resulting mixture thickens, fine. Either way, go to step 4.
4. Pour the mixture into a glass bowl and microwave it for about 11 seconds. Mix vigorously to a creamy consistency. For a double recipe, microwave 16 seconds (approximately, as microwaves vary), mix vigorously, microwave for another 16 seconds, mix again.

NOTE: Delicious served over cooked asparagus.

YIELD: Enough for 2 servings

Eggs Benedict
on Smoked Turkey Hash

Wonderful for brunch on a bleak winter morning, eggs Benedict are warming and filling when served on a hash base. And making hash is the very best way to dispose of the bits of smoked turkey left after you've sliced up the breast. Be sure to add plenty of pepper, some salt, and milk.

    Chopped smoked turkey
    Cooked potatoes, cubed, equal in amount to the turkey
    Milk
    Salt and pepper
    Eggs
    Mexican Mint Hollandaise (see recipe, page 158)

1. Heat the smoked turkey bits and potatoes.
2. Mix in enough milk to produce a hashlike consistency.
3. Season with salt and pepper.
4. Carefully puncture the yolk of each egg (I use a fork) and micro-wave each in a separate bowl. Microwaves differ. Mine does it in 29 seconds.
5. Set each egg on a "nest" of hash.
6. Pour the warm Mexican Mint Hollandaise over each serving.

Mexican Mint Picnic Chicken

Delicious as a main course, this substitutes heat-loving Mexican mint for the original tarragon in a classic chicken dish. This chicken is superb in salad—perfect for a Fourth of July picnic.

    1 large chicken breast (about 2½ pounds), bone in
    6 sprigs of Mexican mint
    1 tablespoon olive oil

1 cup Mexican Mint Dressing (recipe follows)
1 cup seedless grapes, removed from the stems

1. Begin with chicken that is as dry as you can pat it.
2. Carefully loosen the skin on either side of the breastbone to create 2 pockets for the sprigs of Mexican mint.
3. Tuck 3 sprigs into each pocket.
4. Massage the olive oil into the skin.
5. Bake the chicken breast in a 375° oven for 1 hour, or until it is thoroughly cooked. Let stand until cool—about an hour.
6. Discard the skin and sprigs of Mexican mint. Tear the chicken into strips. Toss with the dressing and refrigerate until ready to use.
7. Add the grapes, toss, and serve.

YIELD: 4 servings

Mexican Mint Dressing

½ cup mayonnaise
¼ cup sour cream
3 tablespoons white wine vinegar
3 tablespoons finely chopped Mexican mint, or 1 heaping tablespoon dry
¼ teaspoon dried mustard
¾ teaspoon salt, or to taste
Pepper

1. Combine all the ingredients.
2. Taste for seasoning.
3. Refrigerate until ready to use.

NOTE: Use the remaining dressing for potato salad.

YIELD: 2 cups

Milk Thistle

SILYBUM MARIANUM

BOTANICAL NAME: *Silybum marianum,* Asteraceae.

COMMON NAMES: Milk thistle, Mary's thistle.

DESCRIPTION: Biennial.

Height: To 4 feet.

Flowers: Small fuchsia thistle flowers.

Leaves: Variegated young leaves. Can be cooked and used in salads.

HARVEST: Young leaves; seeds in fall.

CULTURE: Sun, good drainage, ordinary soil.

USE: An outstanding liver tonic.

COMMENTS: Milk thistle may self-sow; in dry climates, it can become a pest. Keep watch for unwanted seedlings.

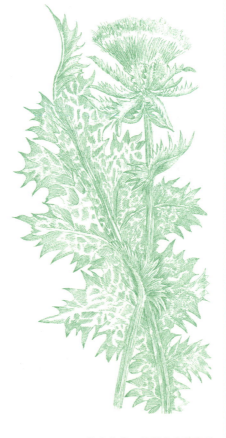

Milk thistle is a big, stately, handsome biennial with stunningly variegated leaves. It was formerly used as a vegetable, and its common name refers to its use in stimulating nursing mothers' production of milk. Today it is invaluable for another of its traditional uses in folk medicine, which is as a general liver tonic. Many people use it as a restorative after drinking alcohol.

Milk thistle comes up easily from seed sown in a sunny place after the ground has warmed in spring; or you can start it in early fall for the following year's garden. Whenever you start it, site milk thistle in a place where you won't have to reach across it or bump into it; it reaches nearly three feet tall by almost as wide. And it is also every bit a thistle—excessively prickly to the touch.

Milk thistle produces dozens of small, purple thistle flowers that are followed by seedpods. Inside these armed receptacles are seeds (technically, fruits) that contain milk thistle's compounds, or silymarin. Silymarin's action is concentrated almost entirely on the liver.

Not only does silymarin support the liver and maintain its normal function, it actually aids the liver in producing new cells. In Europe, silymarin is used to fight liver disease caused by alcoholism and exposure to toxic chemicals. In injectable form silymarin has been used in Germany as an emergency treatment for mushroom poisoning. It has been shown to be effective even in poisoning by *Amanita phalloides*, the deadly mushroom that usually causes irreversible liver damage and death. The German Commission E lists milk thistle as a supportive treatment in chronic inflammation of the liver and cirrhosis.

Nothing short of these miraculous healing properties would make one persevere with milk thistle seedpods. Just one harvest made me want to run screaming to the local health food store for a standardized tincture. Because each lethally spined pod yields only about ⅛ teaspoon (about ¼ gram) of seeds, the going would be slow under any circumstances. Given that the dry pods are the devil's own design, progress is glacial. Dissecting them with bare fingers gets you microscopic tips of thorns embedded in your fingers. Wear gloves or use two tweezers to tear off the prickly layers that encase the hairy choke (as in artichoke).

Each seed—about a quarter of an inch long—is attached to a little tuft of cream-color hairs. When you pull these off, you will have a seed. Many hours later, you should have enough seeds to make a tincture. I ended up with not enough seeds for tincture making to be worthwhile and began thinking about making a tea. According to phytochemical expert Varro E. Tyler, however, "silymarin is very poorly soluble in water, so the herb is not effective in the form of a tea."

Back to square one and tincture making, I bought some milk thistle seeds. The humiliating part was how much larger the store-bought seeds were than the ones I had grown. The recipe below is adapted from the standard recipe for tinctures.

Morning-After Milk Thistle Tonic

Use a food-grade alcohol, 190 proof, available at liquor stores. I tried a mortar and pestle to grind the seeds, quickly gave up, and found that a coffee grinder did the job.

> 1 ounce (or 28 grams) milk thistle seeds (about 50 pods' worth), ground
> 140 milliliters food-grade alcohol

1. Place the ground seeds in the bottom of a jelly jar.
2. Add the alcohol.
3. Seal the jar tightly, shake vigorously, and put it somewhere you won't forget to shake it.
4. Shake the jar once (or twice, if you think of it) daily for 1 month.
5. Use a coffee filter to strain the tincture. Then bottle it. If you save the brown bottles that standardized tinctures come in, you'll also have a dropper to administer the right dose.
6. Store the tincture out of the light.

NOTE: The dose is 1 teaspoonful a day.

Mint

BOTANICAL NAME: *Mentha* spp., Labiatae.

COMMON NAMES: Peppermint, spearmint, pineapple mint, apple mint.

DESCRIPTION: Perennial herb.

Height: To 2 feet.

Flowers: Lavender-pink at the tips of branches.

Leaves: Highly aromatic, gently medicinal; used in cooking.

HARVEST: As needed, or cut mint just as the flower buds start to open. To dry, hang bunches in an airy place, out of the sun. When the bunches are thoroughly dry, strip the leaves from the stems and store them in jars until you are ready to use them.

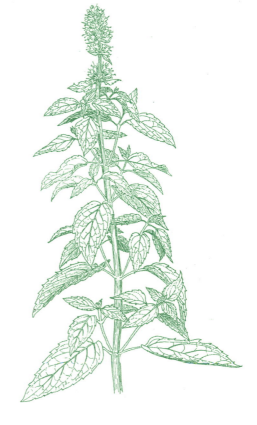

CULTURE: Grow mints in fertile, moist, well-drained soil in sun. Because mints are vigorous plants, they will tolerate shade, but the aroma and essential oil content will not be as concentrated.

USE: Tea from easy-to-grow mints treats nausea, motion sickness, indigestion, and flatulence.

COMMENTS: Buy plants. Mints do not come true from seed.

*Mints are like stray cats; you take them in, give them some food, and they are
yours forever.*
                                                          —Arthur O. Tucker

*T*here are literally dozens of kinds of mints, and probably all of them
have some health benefits. Perhaps the mint most commonly used medicinally is peppermint *(Mentha × piperita)*, a sterile hybrid of spearmint
(Mentha spicata), and water mint *(Mentha aquatica)*. Peppermint contains
menthol. It relieves gas, has an antispasm effect on digestive muscle, and
tends to stimulate the production of bile. It also contains antioxidants
that help prevent age-related diseases. Its oil is effective against *Candida
albicans*—an underlying factor in irritable bowel syndrome—and, as recent research in India suggests, is an effective antifungal agent.

Among the peppermints are the dark-stemmed black peppermints,
often sold as 'Mitcham,' and a form with beautiful dark-chocolate stems
and leaf edges that contrast with the fine green of the leaves that is sold
by nurseries as chocolate mint.

Gently medicinal spearmint *(Mentha spicata)* contains carvone, a digestive. Spearmint is an all-purpose workhorse, used to flavor jellies, teas, and
sauces. Its botanical name *spicata* refers to its long, spiky flower heads.

Pretty pineapple mint *(Mentha suaveolens* 'Variegata') is a strikingly
variegated green and cream. Its green form, apple mint *(Mentha suaveolens)* is the only mint that contains both menthol and carvone. It is great
for teas and cooking.

Start your mint patch with plants or root cuttings. Many mints, including peppermint, do not come true from seed. Grow these perennial
herbs in moist soil in sun or light shade in the ground; they are good
companions to cabbage and tomatoes. Mints grow from eighteen inches
to just over two feet, but when they get scraggly, cut them back to promote fresh new growth.

Mints also make terrific container plants and hanging baskets. Give
them rich soil, fertilizer, and plenty of water.

Most mints are so easy to grow that one of the most commonly
asked questions about their culture is how to contain them. Some people
sink containers into the ground, but it may be easier simply to inspect
the mint patch once or twice during the growing season and use a shovel
to reduce the size of the clump and cut off runaway plants.

One good thing about rampant growth is that it produces plenty of mint. After you use it liberally to flavor fruit salads and tabouli, there will still be plenty left to dry for teas.

Jan's Peppermint Sorbet

This recipe was given to me by Jan Midgley, in whose family it has been used for generations to make a delicious mint syrup for flavoring iced tea. And it does make an excellent flavoring to add to tea—both iced and hot. I loved it as a syrup, but I don't drink much iced tea, so I tried freezing it in my ice-cream maker. As a sorbet, it's nothing short of fabulous.

   2 cups sugar
2½ cups water
     Juice of 6 lemons
     Juice and grated peel of 2 oranges
   4 large handfuls (about 20 sprigs) of peppermint (or mixed mints), washed clean and dried

1. Dissolve the sugar in the water and boil together for 10 minutes.
2. Pour the hot syrup over fruit juices, grated orange peel, and mint.
3. Cover and let steep for several hours.
4. Strain. Allow the mixture to cool before pouring it into an ice-cream maker.
5. Process until frozen.

NOTE: If you prefer to make syrup, pour the mixture into jars and refrigerate. The syrup keeps well for several weeks. Use it in iced tea, mixed drinks, or as a slush.

YIELD: About 24 oz. of syrup; 4 to 6 servings of sorbet

Mint Iced Coffee

Adapted from a recipe published by the Herb Society of Central Indiana, this summer refresher uses low-calorie skim milk, and stevia as the sweetener.

⅓ cup fresh, chopped mint leaves
Freshly ground coffee, enough for 2–4 cups
Ice
1 cup skim milk
1 tablespoon stevia leaves, crumbled

1. Place the mint leaves in the bottom of a coffee press or in the paper basket of an automatic coffeepot. Add the coffee.
2. Make the coffee and allow it to cool to room temperature.
3. Pour into a tall glass filled with ice. Top with milk and stevia, or other sweetener.

YIELD: 2 to 4 servings

> **TIP**
>
> *Mint leaves keep ants away. Strew sprigs of mint in places where ants come in. Or brew up a strong tea and spray.*

Lamb with a Peppermint Crust

If you, like me, have found mint jelly too sweet and minty to go with lamb, this combination of mint, parsley, and garlic in a savory crust might be just subtle enough. Oddly, the inspiration for this recipe came from the many wonderful crusts for quiche in Mollie Katzen's The Enchanted Broccoli Forest, *a vegetarian cookbook.*

> 1 loin roast of lamb, with fat and silver skin removed
> 2 cloves garlic cut into long quarters, plus 2 cloves grated
>   Vegetable oil
> 3 tablespoons bread crumbs (multigrain bread works well)
> 3 tablespoons finely chopped fresh peppermint
> 1 tablespoon finely chopped parsley
> ¼ teaspoon salt
>   Pepper
>   Olive oil

1. Preheat the oven to 350°.
2. Make deep cuts into the lamb and insert the slivers of garlic.
3. Truss the lamb and sear it in the vegetable oil. Allow it to cool.
4. Mix the bread crumbs, peppermint, parsley, grated garlic, salt, and pepper with just enough olive oil to make a paste.
5. Spread the mixture over the lamb. Place the lamb in the oven.
6. Roast for 20 minutes per pound.

YIELD: 8 servings

Indiana Cold Mint Pea Salad

The state of Indiana is ranked third to fifth in the world (depending upon the season) for spearmint production and fourth in the production of peppermint. This recipe comes from the Herb Society of Central Indiana—cooks who know a thing or two about mint. Mint is a strong flavor. You may wish to try the recipe once with half the amount of mint.

2 bags (10 ounces) frozen peas

½ cup light sour cream

6 green onions, chopped

¼ cup chopped fresh mint (apple mint would be nice), plus additional leaves for garnish

⅓ cup cooked bacon bits

Salt and pepper

1. Thaw and drain the peas.
2. Combine all the ingredients except the whole mint leaves. Chill.
3. Garnish with mint leaves and serve.

YIELD: 8 servings

TIP

To preserve flavor and fragrance, add fresh mint to hot foods at the end of cooking.

Steep mint in warm milk (½ to 1 cup) when making custards, sauces, or ice cream. Strain the milk before using and discard the mint.

Mugwort

ARTEMISIA VULGARIS

BOTANICAL NAME: *Artemisia vulgaris,* Asteraceae.

COMMON NAMES: Mugwort, *moxa* (Chinese).

DESCRIPTION: Perennial.

Height: To 6 feet.

Flowers: Small spikes of blue flowers between the leaves at the ends of branches; they appear in July and August.

Leaves: Toothed leaves are green above and silvery white below.

HARVEST: Cut and dry the whole plant as needed for dream pillows or, in fall, for use in dried arrangements and wreaths.

CULTURE: Zones 3 to 10. Grows in sun and poor soil; needs drainage.

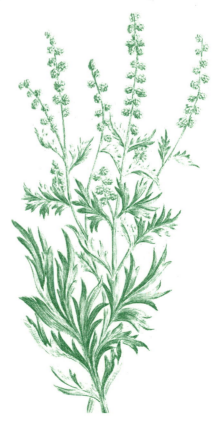

USE: Mugwort is used in acupuncture; for stimulating dreams; and in dried arrangements. It can become a pest in the garden.

COMMENTS: Mugwort may help some people to sleep.

OTHER SPECIES: French tarragon (*Artemisia dracunculus* var. *sativa*) for cooking; wormwood (*Artemisia absinthium)* for intestinal worms, liver; *Artemisia lactiflora* for liver disorders; sweet annie *(Artemisia annua)* for malaria.

*U*sed in Ayurvedic medicine for gynecological problems and fungal infections, mugwort is known in China as *moxa* and is used in acupuncture. Traditionally, a bundle of smoldering compressed mugwort is applied to an acupuncture point. In this country, the practice is modified: cigar-like bundles of the leaves are burned and held close to or on the needle to add heat.

Like St.-John's-wort, mugwort has been linked with superstition and legend since medieval times. Garlands and crowns of mugwort were thought to ward off evil spirits and witches. A pillow filled with mugwort was thought to stimulate dreams.

The idea of stimulating dreams had such great appeal that I made a mugwort pillow to take to bed. It was during a troubled period in which I suffered from insomnia. I reasoned that because the sense of smell is directly linked to the brain, it might well work. If I could write down my dreams, I might confront the subconscious in my waking hours. What I found was that when I slept with the mugwort pillow, my sleep was deep and uninterrupted. If there were dreams, I couldn't remember them upon waking.

Mugwort is so easy to grow in almost any soil and sun conditions that it has naturalized everywhere, and it may become a pest in your garden as well as in ditches and other waste places. If you can't find a plant, grow it from seed (see Sources).

It grows tremendously in its first year in the garden, and it may reach six feet in subsequent years. Mugwort, with leaves that are green above and silver below, is a beautiful addition to fresh and dried flower bouquets and wreathes. A variegated form, *Artemisia vulgaris* 'Variegata,' is often seen in nurseries.

Other species of *Artemisia* figure in culinary and medicinal gardens. First among these is French tarragon (*Artemisia dracunculus* var. *sativa*), whose minty anise-like flavor is essential in cooking. Among the wormwoods, *Artemisia absinthium,* now outlawed as a flavoring for absinthe liqueur because it caused damage to the nervous system in habitual drinkers, is still used for short-term treatment of intestinal worms and for a liver tonic. *Artemisia lactiflora,* white mugwort, which adorns gardens with its bold habit and astilbe-like flowers, is used in China as a remedy for liver disorders.

Artemisia annua, sweet annie, has been in the news lately. Found to destroy malarial parasites, it can be successful in treating drug-resistant malaria. In Chinese medicine, it is called *qing hao* and has a long history of use for fevers and night sweats.

Long Creek Herbs Sleep Pillow

I made a sleep pillow by combining equal parts dried mugwort and lavender and encasing them in a muslin bag. That was before Jim Long, author of Making Herbal Dream Pillows, *shared his recipe with me. His business, Long Creek Herbs, sells all kinds of sleep pillows (see Sources). Jim Long says that this mixture has worked for Vietnam vets who suffer from flashbacks and nightmares. This recipe makes enough for several pillows.*

¼ cup dried lavender flower buds
¼ cup dried mugwort
¼ cup dried sweet hops
¼ cup dried roses

Combine all the ingredients. To make one pillow, put about 2 tablespoons of the mix into a little pillow covering or muslin bag, or "even an old sock that's clean." Tuck the little pillow into your pillowcase. It doesn't matter where it goes. Sleep easy!

Mullein

BOTANICAL NAME: *Verbascum thapsus,* Scrophulariaceae.

COMMON NAMES: Mullein, great mullein, Aaron's rod, flannel plant.

DESCRIPTION: Biennial.

> *Height:* To 6 feet.

> *Flowers:* Yellow in a terminal spike.

> *Leaves:* Large, downy, gray, in a basal rosette.

HARVEST: Cut whole plants when they flower; dry leaves and flowers to use in infusions and tinctures. The flowers are used in oil for a chest rub.

CULTURE: Zones 5 to 9; easy; sun to part shade, ordinary soil.

USE: For coughs and upper respiratory infections, and as a very mild sedative.

COMMENTS: Self-sows with a vengeance.

OTHER SPECIES:

> *V. densiflorum* has similar medicinal properties.

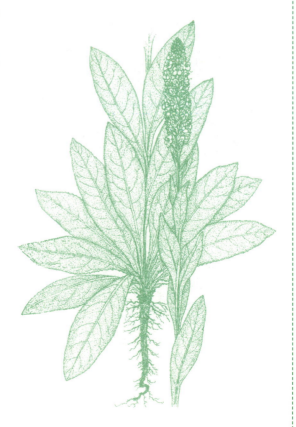

*M*ullein arrived in my garden one fine spring day—an uninvited but very welcome guest. Now its descendants are scattered throughout the garden. The first-year plants of this biennial herb almost never need transplanting or removal. Low, gray-green rosettes of fuzzy leaves adorn their sites like big bows.

In the second year, however, mullein sends up a 6-to-8-foot flower stalk that is handsome in the back of a border but a nuisance in a path. Nevertheless, the flowers as well as the leaves are medicinally valuable.

Mullein has a tradition dating to classical times as a remedy for upper respiratory ailments. It is on the German Commission E's list for catarrh and upper respiratory complaints. In Colonial America, leaves were smoked and taken in a tea for coughs and tuberculosis. Thick and flannel-like, they also served as insulation in socks to keep feet warm, and they were used as diapers.

A simple and effective remedy for congestion and hacking coughs is mullein tea, made by steeping one tablespoon of dried mullein—leaves and flowers—in eight ounces of boiled water for ten minutes. Sweeten with honey or Jan's Peppermint Syrup (see Jan's Peppermint Sorbet, page 166). It should be drunk twice daily.

If you are not especially prone to coughs and colds, combine the dried flowers in a sleep tea along with other calming herbs such as chamomile, peppermint, gotu kola, and lemon verbena. Taking this tea is a pleasant bedtime ritual that ensures deep, restorative sleep.

Serene Slumber Tea

Very pleasing and effective.

    ½ cup dried mullein flowers
    ½ cup dried chamomile flowers
    2 tablespoons dried gotu kola leaves
    2 tablespoons dried peppermint leaves
    2 tablespoons dried lemon verbena

1. Combine the herbs. Store in a covered tin. Mix before each use, because the finer pieces settle at the bottom.
2. To use, pour 8 ounces boiling water over 1 tablespoon herb mixture. Allow to steep for 10 minutes. Sweeten to taste.

Nettle

URTICA DIOICA

BOTANICAL NAME: *Urtica dioica,* Urticaceae.

COMMON NAMES: Nettle, stinging nettle.

DESCRIPTION: Perennial.

Height: To 6 feet.

Flowers: Inconspicuous, greenish flowers appear in early summer.

Leaves: Edible when dried or cooked. Leaves are armed with stinging hairs when fresh.

HARVEST: Young leaves for greens or tea; the whole plant for an excellent organic fertilizer.

CULTURE: Zones 4 to 8. Very easy; sun to part shade, moist, well-drained soil.

USE: Tonic, cystitis tea; nutrient-rich green; organic fertilizer.

COMMENTS: Very aggressive; keep it away from small, fragile herbs that may be engulfed.

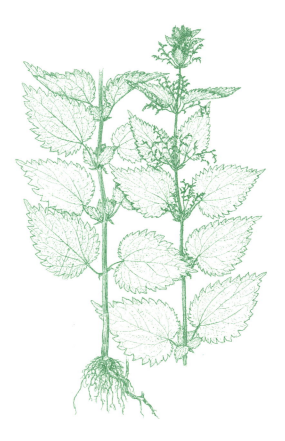

*F*irst the bad news: stinging nettle is aptly named. When you touch nettle, bristly hairs along the leaves and stems break off, releasing formic acid that stings and causes red bumps to form on the skin.

The good news is that once nettle is dried or cooked, it doesn't sting. You can use gloves to harvest its amazing nutritional richness. Loaded with minerals—including calcium, magnesium, potassium, selenium, and zinc—nettle also contains over 25 percent protein. Rich in vitamins A and C, it was once used to prevent scurvy, and it is a folk remedy for arthritis.

Today nettle aids in healing allergies, particularly those of the upper respiratory system. Along with cranberries or blueberries, it is an excellent remedy for cystitis. On the German Commission E's approved list for irrigation therapy for inflammation of the lower urinary tract, it is also used to prevent kidney gravel. When drunk as a tea, nettle also acts as a general tonic.

Not only is this green vegetable nutritious, it virtually grows itself and is available when little else is around to harvest. Nettle comes up quickly from seed started in the garden or inside on a sunny windowsill. And once it gets going in the garden, it's hard to stop. It is a perennial that spreads by both rhizomes and seeds.

When a plant exceeds its space, you can trim the rhizomes with a spade and plant them elsewhere to enlarge your patch. Or you can recycle these nitrogen-rich greens, adding valuable hot material to your compost.

Harvesting is not difficult, but it requires precautions: gloves and, perhaps, long sleeves and pants. (If, in spite of all precautions, you get stung, rub the skin with the crushed leaf of mullein or jewelweed.) The parts to harvest for greens are the tender top growths and leaves not much larger than an inch long.

Nettle grows fast; before you know it, your plants will grow big and rank. Whenever this happens, cut nettle back to the ground and save the plants for compost or nettle fertilizer (see below). The cut-back plants will send up new shoots with delicate young leaves, keeping a succession of edible greens coming. Combine nettle with other greens (see Jan Midgley's Classic Greens recipe, page 66).

Although they are not tender enough for greens, the big leaves you cut back are also useful for tea. Hang them in bunches in an airy place, out of direct sun. When they are thoroughly dry, strip the leaves, pack them into jars, and store out of the light.

Nettle Tea

A tea made with fresh or dried nettle leaves will purify the blood and keep cystitis at bay. Drink it two or three times each day. It doesn't taste like much. Honey is a necessity—or add Jan's mint syrup (see Jan's Peppermint Sorbet, page 166).

    1 cup boiling water
    ½ cup fresh nettle leaves, or 4 teaspoons dried
      Honey

1. Pour boiling water over the leaves and allow to steep for 10 minutes.
2. Strain. Sweeten to taste with honey.

YIELD: 1 serving

Nettle-Flecked Parsnips and Turnips

An accidental combination, this mixture is pretty and delicious.

    2 cups chopped turnips (2)
    2 cups chopped parsnips (2 large)
    1 cup water (more or less)
    1 cup nettle leaves
    1 tablespoon butter
    ½ teaspoon salt plus additional to taste
      Pepper

1. In a 2-quart saucepan, combine the turnips and parsnips and just enough water to keep the vegetables from sticking. Cook until soft, about 15 minutes.

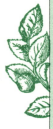

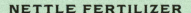

NETTLE FERTILIZER

When you've harvested enough nettle for your own use, put the rest to work in the garden. Rich in nutrients, nettle plants are terrific additions to a compost heap and make a wonderful fertilizing tea.

1. Cut old and tough nettle stems and foliage down to the ground and place in a plastic bucket. Cover with water (rainwater is great, if you can catch it).
2. Add other herbs such as tansy, comfrey, dandelion, and horsetail, if available.
3. Mix every day. The tea will soon smell very bad—a good sign.
4. Wait 3 weeks or so, until fermentation has ceased.
5. Dilute with water at a ratio of 1:10 and apply to the soil in the vegetable garden.

2. Add the nettle leaves and cook about 3 minutes, or until they are very wilted.
3. Add the butter and ½ teaspoon of the salt and mash with a potato masher or a fork. The mixture should be lumpy but well mixed.
4. Add salt and pepper to taste.

NOTE: This is a delicious and attractive accompaniment for pork chops.

YIELD: 4 servings

Nettle Soup

Nettle is an important green in Ireland, Scotland, and Scandinavia. I found any number of recipes for nettle soup in cookbooks from these countries, but in the end concocted my own version. Of the many forays into the making of nettle soup, this one was the tastiest.

    1 leek, cut into ½-inch rounds
    2 tablespoons olive oil
    1½ cups young nettle leaves
    1½ cups squash (such as zucchini)
       Salt and pepper
    2 cups chicken broth

1. Saute the leek in the olive oil until it is soft.
2. Add the nettle leaves and squash. Season with salt and pepper and cook for another 5 to 10 minutes.
3. Add the chicken broth and cook until all the vegetables are very soft, about 15 minutes.
4. Blend. Serve hot or cold.

YIELD: 4 servings

Onion

ALLIUM SPP.

BOTANICAL NAME: *Allium* spp., Liliaceae.

COMMON NAME: Onion.

DESCRIPTION: Bulbs.

> *Height:* To 24 inches.
>
> *Flowers:* Cut off when buds form.
>
> *Leaves:* Edible, long, narrow.

HARVEST: As needed. For storage, bend the tops over when they turn yellow; dig the bulbs when the tops are dry. Cure.

CULTURE: Sow seed or plant onion sets in sun, in well-drained, light, fertile loam enriched with a balanced fertilizer (raised beds are excellent); lime if your soil has a pH below 6. Plant cloves in fall, with their pointed ends up, and about a half inch below the soil surface. In cold climates, provide a winter mulch. Grow near lettuce, peppers, and dill.

USE: Delicious blood-thinners that improve circulation and digestion.

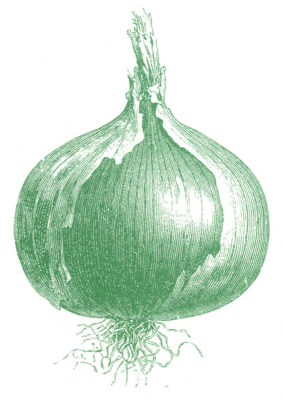

COMMENTS: Eat onions every day.

OTHER SPECIES: Shallot *(Allium ascalonicum)*; shallot greens make tasty scallions. The nodding onion *(Allium cernuum)*, a native ornamental, yields lovely pink, edible flowers for salads and garnish.

*O*nions are a given in cooking, an absolute essential. So it is gratifying to find that something you already enjoy eating has medicinal properties. The next time you fix a bowl of onion soup, think of it as therapy for the circulatory, digestive, and respiratory systems.

Red and yellow onions are a rich source of quercetin, a natural substance that has been shown to suppress the growth of certain cancer cells. They may contain up to 10 percent of their dry weight as quercetin—a boon for enthusiastic onion eaters, who enjoy a lower incidence of certain types of cancer.

White onions contain little or no quercetin, which is not to say that they are worthless nutritionally. Other compounds in all onions help thin the blood, lower cholesterol, and prevent arteriosclerosis (for which use they are included on the German Commission E's approved list). There are many different kinds of onions. What grows well in one part of the country may not do so in another. Of all the onions, my choice is a near relative—shallots. I like to use them in cooking, and I grow them because they are so expensive to buy.

I bought two types of shallots to plant: a classic French gray and a yellow multiplier type that falls somewhere between shallots and onions in character. Although the rotund yellow multipliers produced a larger harvest, I preferred the hard, narrower, tear-shaped French shallots for their taste and longevity.

When you buy shallots for planting, you get whole bulbs that have to be divided—ever so gently—into cloves. Plant the cloves in fall, pushing each one into the soil, pointy end up, until it is a half inch or so beneath the surface and a foot from other cloves in all directions. Each clove will produce a whole new bulb. Yellow multipliers produced more than one bulb.

One year, when I was running late, I forgot to plant the shallots until very late winter and was surprised at how well and how quickly they produced. But that was a mild winter in the Mid-Atlantic region. If you live in the northern parts of the country, fall planting is safer.

Shallots and onions are ready when their tops turn yellow, although you can harvest them sooner if there is need. Hold back on watering as the plants reach maturity, because the bulbs need dry conditions to form their protective skins. When the tops flop over, dig the bulbs carefully and cure them.

Curing Shallots and Onions

1. After digging shallots or onions, spread them out in the sun for a day, until the roots dry up.
2. Use a drying rack (a screen raised to allow for air beneath works very well, but I've also used a slatted wooden table) in an airy, covered place to dry them.
3. Wait until the neck of the onion is tight and the skin flaky. Then trim the tops to 8 inches and braid them into chains to hang in a cool room. Or you can trim the tops to 1 inch and store the shallots or onions in net shopping bags or netted onion bags (see Sources).

Shallot Butter

Butters are a great way to add the taste of herbs or, in this case, shallots to whatever you are cooking. Make enough to have some on hand without all the peeling and chopping. Use on everything—beef, chicken, vegetables.

½ cup unsalted butter
2 tablespoons finely minced shallots
¼ teaspoon salt, optional

1. Using a mortar and pestle, soften the butter.
2. Blend in the shallots and, if using, the salt.

Parsley

PETROSELINUM CRISPUM 'ITALIAN PLAIN LEAF' VAR. *NEOPOLITANUM*

BOTANICAL NAME: *Petroselinum crispum* var. *neopolitanum,* Apiaceae.

COMMON NAME: Parsley.

DESCRIPTION: Biennial.

> *Height:* To 15 inches.
>
> *Flowers:* White umbels in the second summer.
>
> *Leaves:* Edible, flavorful, indispensable in cooking.

HARVEST: As needed.

CULTURE: Grow parsley in sun to part shade in well-drained soil.

USE: A gentle blood purifier; an aid to digestion; a breath and palate cleanser; an important flavoring.

COMMENTS: Parsley attracts the light green and black caterpillars of the swallowtail butterfly. It's nice to have several extra parsley plants to share with these lovely creatures.

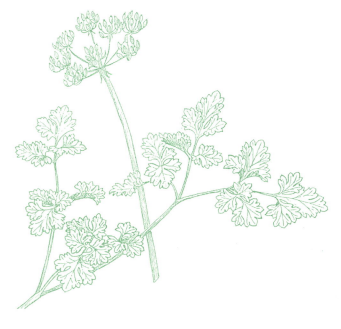

*A*ll too often, the parsley on our plates is merely a garnish and not intended to be eaten. That's a terrible waste of a gently medicinal and flavorful culinary herb. Rich in vitamins A and C, niacin, riboflavin, and calcium, parsley clears the body of toxins, reduces inflammation, and aids in digestion—to say nothing of its palate- and breath-cleansing actions. According to *The Complete Book of Natural & Medicinal Cures*, from the editors of Prevention Magazine Health Books, dried parsley concentrates the minerals: "Gram for gram, it provides two to three times more copper, iron, magnesium, and boron than almost any other food."

Parsley herb and root are on the German Commission E's list of safe and efficacious medicinal herbs. Used crushed in infusions, parsley is helpful in flushing out the urinary tract, and it prevents kidney gravel.

Parsley is pretty—as attractive in the garden as it is on the plate. It is just the right size—about fifteen inches tall—to edge a garden bed. A biennial, parsley greens up early in the spring of its second year and makes a stunning companion to pansies. At about midsummer, it will flower, go to seed, and die. You can keep it going longer as an ornamental if you continue to pinch off the flower stalk, but the flavor becomes bitter, making the parsley useless for cooking.

Or, for an endless supply of parsley, replant it every year as an annual and enjoy the bonus of second-year parsley in spring.

Parsley also grows well on a windowsill from seeds started around midsummer. Soak the seeds overnight before planting them directly in clean pots of sterile potting mix with a one-inch layer of seed starter mix on top (these mixtures are available at garden centers and hardware stores). Keep the soil moist until seedlings appear. Acclimate the young plants slowly to conditions of lower light before bringing them indoors. For example, start the seedlings in full sun. Once they've started active growth, remove the pot first into part shade and then into full shade before bringing it inside.

> ## TIP
>
> *Parsley is good for you. Eat it in salads. Keep some sprigs in a vase of water in the kitchen and sprinkle it chopped over almost everything.*

Kamut with Parsley
and Onion Greens

Kamut is an ancient rice with great big nutty-tasting grains. It's a delicious change from ordinary white rice and goes well with assertive flavors like those of parsley and onions. This recipe is basically an adaptation of the "green rice" idea that's been around kitchens forever, but instead of spinach I used parsley and onion greens, and instead of white rice I used kamut.

> 1 cup kamut or other rice
> 6–8 onion-family greens (chives, shallot greens, or green
>   onions)
> 1 tablespoon olive oil
>   Salt and pepper
> 3 tablespoons finely chopped parsley
> ¾ cup toasted pecan pieces

1. Cook the kamut according to the directions on the package or about one and one-half times as long as rice.
2. Fry the onion greens in the olive oil. Season with salt and pepper and add to the kamut.
3. Mix in the parsley.
4. Toast the pecan pieces, toss them into the kamut, and serve.

YIELD: 4 servings

Parsley Butter

When you buy a bunch of parsley for a particular dish, there's usually some left over. Put it to good use in this delicious butter. Melt it over noodles or starchy vegetables such as potatoes or turnips. There is no hard-and-fast rule for making herb butters. You can try whatever herbs you have in the garden. Basil is a great ingredient to combine with parsley. And adventuresome souls may mix in garlic for a more assertive flavor.

½ pound butter
1 tablespoon finely chopped Italian parsley
1 tablespoon finely chopped chives
¼ teaspoon lemon juice
¼ teaspoon salt (or to taste)

1. Allow the butter to soften, but not to melt.
2. Add the chopped herbs and mix well.
3. Add the lemon juice and salt. Mix again.
4. Pack into a small glass dish, cover, and refrigerate until ready to use.

François Dionot's Cold Fresh Herb Soup

Students in François Dionot's classes at Washington's l'Academie de Cuisine sometimes gasp at the richness of eggs and cream in the dishes he creates. To those with the temerity to ask about substituting lower-calorie ingredients for this very rich soup, Dionot patiently explains that the amount of cream each person will ultimately consume is relatively small. With a Gallic shrug, he suggests, "Keep the portions small." Why substitute lesser ingredients when serving something absolutely delicious in a small amount accomplishes the same end? To serve this soup, he uses tiny, 2-ounce espresso cups. To "distract the eye" and enlarge the experience, he tops each serving with crème frâiche and a spot of caviar.

1 quart chicken stock
1 cup parsley (or 1 bunch)
1 cup fresh tarragon or Mexican mint (or 1 bunch)
1½ cups basil (or 1 bunch)
Salt and pepper
6 egg yolks
1 cup heavy cream
Ice for cooling the soup
Crème frâiche for garnish
Caviar for garnish

1. Bring the chicken stock to a boil, uncovered, and reduce by half.
2. Meanwhile, chop most of the herbs, keeping the nicer leaves for decoration.

3. When the stock is reduced, bring it down to a simmer and add the herbs. Simmer for 1 minute, then turn off the heat. Steep for 10 minutes.

4. Pass the herbs and stock through a sieve and discard the herbs. Season the stock.

5. Reheat the stock.

6. Mix the egg yolks and cream together.

7. Temper the egg yolk mixture by swiftly mixing in a little of the hot stock. Then pour the mixture into the stock, stirring constantly with a wooden spoon, over medium heat, until the soup thickens enough to coat the back of the spoon. Do not boil. Keep a sieve handy should lumps form.

8. Transfer the soup to a stainless steel bowl and set the bowl in a container of ice. Allow the soup to cool. Season with salt and pepper.

9. Serve the soup cold, garnished with fresh herbs, crème frâiche, and caviar.

YIELD: 16 2-ounce servings

Joan Aghevli's Persian Rice

Joan Aghevli grew up in Australia, but she has learned to cook her husband's favorite Persian dishes. Excellent with grilled or baked fish, this rice uses masses of parsley, along with dill, cilantro, and saffron. Serve it with Joan's Mast-O-Khiar, page 208, a yogurt dish. The idea is to turn out the rice like a cake with a rich, orange crust on top. This is accomplished by turning the pan over with a serving dish underneath to catch the "cake." It doesn't always work. No matter: You can break the crust into pieces and stir it into the rice for a pretty and delicious dish.

   2 cups basmati rice
     Salted water for boiling the rice
  ½ cup butter
   3 cloves garlic, crushed
   2 tablespoons plain yogurt
  ½ teaspoon saffron, ground and dissolved in 1 tablespoon hot water

2½ cups chopped parsley
½ cup chopped scallions
1½ cups chopped dill
1 cup chopped coriander
1 teaspoon ground cinnamon

1. Rinse the rice well in a colander under cold running water.
2. Bring a large pot of salted water to a boil, add the rice, stir, and boil for 8 minutes.
3. Drain the rice into a colander and rinse well under cold running water.
4. In a large nonstick saucepan, melt half of the butter. Add the crushed garlic.
5. In a small bowl, combine 2 big spoonfuls of the rice with the yogurt and a little saffron water. Spoon this mixture evenly over the melted butter.
6. Add the remaining rice and the herbs except the cinnamon to the pot in alternating layers, 2 large spoonfuls of rice to 1 of herbs.
7. Mound the rice and herbs and sprinkle with the cinnamon. Place the pot over medium heat and cook for 10 minutes. Pour the remaining butter and saffron water over the rice mixture.
8. Place three sheets of paper towel or a clean dish towel over the pot and cover firmly with the lid. Reduce the heat to low and cook for 50 minutes. Remove from the heat and let stand for 5 minutes.
9. Stir the remaining saffron and butter gently into the rice; remove a few tablespoons for decorating the rice. At this point, you can try inverting the pan onto a serving platter. With luck, the whole thing will pop out like a cake with a crust on top (do it over a baking sheet just in case). If that doesn't work, break up the crust and stir it into the rice.

YIELD: 8 servings

Pepper

CAPSICUM SPP.

BOTANICAL NAME: *Capsicum* spp., Solanaceae.

COMMON NAMES: Pepper, chili pepper.

DESCRIPTION: Annual.

Height: 18 to 30 inches.

Flowers: Small white, sometimes tinged with lavender, with yellow centers.

Leaves: Green; on hot pepper plants, often tinged with purple; on stiff stems.

HARVEST: The fruits are edible peppers. Wait until red chili peppers turn red to pick. They will have twice the amount of vitamin C as when green.

CULTURE: Slow to germinate, peppers require very warm conditions to germinate and grow.

USE: An excellent source of antiviral, vitamin-rich nutrients; good for colds. Capsaicin in peppers inhibits pain transmitter.

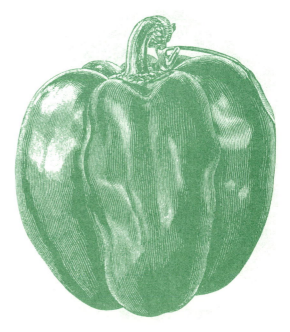

COMMENTS: Wash your hands after handling hot peppers. Be careful not to touch your eyes. To relieve a burning sensation on your hands, dip them in a dilute solution of household bleach in water. And don't overdo eating hot peppers! Too many hot peppers can burn the lining of the stomach. To relieve burning in your mouth, drink milk or eat yogurt.

*I*t isn't only flavor that hot peppers deliver. The fiery taste that beads sweat on your upper lip is capsaicin. It is a substance that has been shown to inhibit the herpes virus and prevent ulcers and cluster headaches. It also blocks the pain of shingles, arthritis, and rheumatism by depleting some of the body's substance P, necessary in pain transmission. Cayenne, derived from hot peppers, figures on the German Commission E's approved list for painful muscle spasms.

Sweet peppers, on the other hand, are loaded with vitamin C. And all peppers—both sweet and hot—are outstanding sources of A, B_1, C, and beta-carotene. Adding them to salads, soups, and stews is a most delicious way to stay healthy.

If I find myself or someone else coming down with a cold, in addition to administering regular doses of zinc and echinacea, I make a hot and spicy chicken soup using plenty of hot peppers.

There are dozens of peppers to choose from: sweet, hot, and all degrees in between. If you want to go gently into pepper cultivation, 'Hungarian Paprika' is a sweet pepper with a hint of heat—an excellent type for drying. You can grind it into your own paprika or simply crumble it into whatever you are cooking. Or try 'Mulato Isleno,' which is a few degrees spicier.

Among the hot peppers are the super-hots, 'Habanero' and 'Thai Hot,' and the classics, 'Jalapeno' and 'Cayenne.' Starting your own pepper plants from seed will give you far greater choice than what you are likely to find as plants at your local nursery center.

Peppers grow best in hot weather. If you are starting them from seed inside for later transplanting into the garden, use peat pellets and set them in your sunniest window. Don't start them too early or they'll be all grown up with nowhere to go. Their ideal germination temperature is between 75 and 85 degrees Fahrenheit, which is easier to maintain with a little help from the spring sun. Also, peppers grow best with plenty of room to spread outward. Starting them early may mean having to pot them up one or more times before they can safely go into the garden.

Wait until late spring, when the soil temperature is at least 65 degrees Fahrenheit, before transplanting them into the garden. Don't mulch until midsummer when the soil is very warm.

Hot and Spicy Chicken Soup

Got a cold? Try this simple soup that combines good-for-you ingredients. I always keep garlic, dried hot peppers, and ginger next to the stove, so this recipe came about naturally. It works wonders for clearing stuffy heads and is clear enough not to put off ailing appetites. Also, the next time you stir-fry, try braising vegetables in a small amount of this soup, instead. Onions, broccoli spears, carrot sticks, and shiitake mushrooms are delicious done this way.

2 cups chicken stock, or 1 can (15 ounces) chicken broth
   1-inch piece of ginger, peeled and sliced
3 cloves (or more) of garlic, peeled, mashed, rested
   Chili peppers, deseeded and broken (or cut, if fresh) into pieces
   (the heat is up to you)
   Salt and pepper

1. Combine all the ingredients in a saucepan.
2. Simmer, covered, for at least 30 minutes.
3. Season with salt and pepper.

YIELD: 3 to 4 servings

> ## TIP
>
> *Keep a few dried chili peppers within reach of your stove. Crumble some chili pepper into just about anything that you cook.*

Queensdale Spicy Pepper Marinade

Barbara Burgess, chef at Queensdale, a bed-and-breakfast in Hillsborough, North Carolina, says that the fire of this versatile marinade depends upon the type of chili pepper used. Delicious as a marinade for shrimp, it is fine as a dressing to toss with shredded cabbage and carrots.

1 tablespoon honey
½ cup balsamic vinegar
1 teaspoon finely grated ginger
½ teaspoon finely grated garlic
    Dried hot pepper, finely ground
½ cup olive oil
1 teaspoon salt (or to taste)
    Freshly ground black pepper

1. Combine the honey and vinegar in a bowl. Whisk together.
2. Stir in the ginger, then the garlic. Then add the red pepper.
3. Whisk in the oil as you add it in a fine stream.
4. Season with salt and pepper.

NOTE: Make this marinade up to a day ahead and store it in a jar in the fridge. Shake hard before using.

YIELD: 1¼ cups

Grilled Marinated Vegetables

Marilyn MacQueen's Queensdale bed-and-breakfast in Hillsborough, North Carolina, is justly famous for its grilled meats and vegetables. An hour or two in the marinade renders these vegetables extraordinary. Served with couscous, they compose a light summer supper or a great accompaniment to grilled meats.

1 sweet pepper, cut into 1-inch slices
1 eggplant, cut into ½-inch slices

1 zucchini, cut into ½-inch slices

1 red onion, cut into ½-inch slices

3 carrots, cut in quarters lengthwise, then into 3- to 4-inch pieces
    Queensdale Spicy Pepper Marinade (see recipe above)

1. Put the vegetables into a bowl; add ½ cup of the marinade.
2. Marinate vegetables for 1 to 3 hours.
3. Grill the vegetables.

YIELD: 6 to 8 servings

Pumpkin

CUCURBITA PEPO

BOTANICAL NAME: *Cucurbita pepo,* Cucurbitaceae.

COMMON NAME: Pumpkin.

DESCRIPTION: Annual.

> *Height:* To 12 inches.

> *Flowers:* Large, yellow; may be eaten.

> *Leaves:* Large, hairy; on extensive vines.

HARVEST: As needed after the pumpkins turn orange, or just before the first frost.

CULTURE: Pumpkins will respond to rich soil and even moisture with larger yields and fruit. If space is limited, grow them on the southern or western edge of the vegetable garden and let them spill over into the lawn.

USE: These highly nutritious fruits are excellent for soups, breads, pies, and as a vegetable. They contain antioxidants.

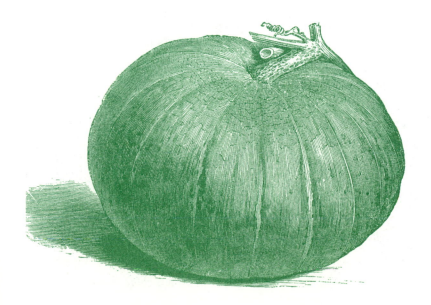

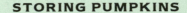

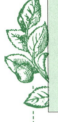

When we hear the word "pumpkin" we usually think of the great big Halloween jack-o'-lantern types. Less daunting to the cook and more prolific are the smaller pumpkins. 'New England Pie,' 'Small Sugar,' 'Baby Bear,' and the French heirloom 'Cinderella' pumpkin, also known as 'Rouge Vif d'Étampes,' are a just few varieties that will delight the cook and fortify those who eat them.

Pumpkin's beta-carotene count is off the chart: just a half cup of cooked pumpkin contains between one and a half to two and a half times the daily recommended amount. In addition to beta-carotene, pumpkin contains other antioxidants and iron. And that's just the flesh of the pumpkin. The seeds are rich in iron and have more protein than an equal weight of meat. They are also rich in zinc, a mineral useful in treating enlarged prostate. Pumpkin seeds—either whole or coarsely ground—are on the German Commission E's approved list to treat irritated bladder and problems of benign prostate hyperplasia, stages 1 and 2.

Accidental Curried Pumpkin Soup

This great Thanksgiving soup is beautiful, orange, and hot and spicy. It was the result of my going on dopey autopilot when too much was going on around me—

twelve for dinner, kids home from school, dog jumping the fence. I'd planned to use sweet potato as the base for a soup, but when the time came to cook, there wasn't enough. There was, however, a little pumpkin from the garden. The result was this warming, filling soup, rich in vitamin A and potassium for healthy skin.

1 tablespoon olive oil
2 tablespoons Curry in a Hurry (page 58)
1 tablespoon curry powder
2 cups pumpkin, peeled and cut into chunks (see note)
1 large sweet potato, cut into chunks
4 cups chicken stock
1 cinnamon stick (5 inches)
   Salt and pepper
1 cube good-quality chicken bouillon (if necessary)

1. Heat the olive oil and add the Curry in a Hurry, cooking for 3 to 4 minutes.
2. Add the curry powder, stir together, and cook another 3 minutes or so. The mixture will darken to brown.
3. Add the pumpkin, sweet potato, broth, and cinnamon stick. Simmer until tender, about 30 minutes.
4. Allow the soup to cool before removing the cinnamon stick and blending the soup in batches.
5. Taste for seasoning and add salt and pepper. If the flavor is weak, add a bouillon cube and blend again.

NOTE: A small pumpkin (8 inches in diameter) provides about 4 cups of pumpkin—enough to double this recipe or make Pumpkin Bread with Pepitas (recipe follows).

YIELD: 12 servings

TIP

To make a pumpkin easier to peel, stab several holes in it, place it in the microwave, and cook for about 10 minutes. Wait until it is cool enough to handle, then cut it into chunks and peel.

Pumpkin Bread with Pepitas

I've lost touch with Ellen Seale, who gave me this recipe when our children attended the Garret Park Cooperative Nursery School, but I've thought of her a hundred times as I cooked this bread over the years. It keeps well and is ideal for packing up and shipping to college dorms. It has garnered fans at three colleges.

   3 cups sugar
   1 cup oil
   4 eggs, beaten
   2 cups cooked pumpkin, or 1 can (16 ounces)
   ⅔ cup water
   1 teaspoon baking powder
   2 teaspoons baking soda
   2 teaspoons salt
   ¼ teaspoon cloves
   1 teaspoon cinnamon
   1 teaspoon nutmeg
   1 teaspoon allspice
   3½ cups flour
      Pepitas (hulled pumpkin seeds) for topping

1. Preheat the oven to 350°.
2. Mix together all of the ingredients except the flour and the pepitas.
3. Add the flour; mix.
4. Top with pepitas and bake in three loaf pans for one hour.

YIELD: 3 loaves, 8 servings each

Purslane

PORTULACA OLERACEA SATIVA

BOTANICAL NAME: *Portulaca oleracea sativa,* Portulaceae.

COMMON NAME: Purslane.

DESCRIPTION: Annual.

Height: 2 to 12 inches.

Flowers: Small, yellow.

Leaves: Thickened, succulent, spoon-shaped, on reddish stems.

HARVEST: Before flowers appear; regular removal of new growth stimulates more growth. For use as a green vegetable, cut the whole plant to within 1 inch of the ground.

CULTURE: Sow in late spring, early summer. Grow in sun, in ordinary soil.

USE: Source of antioxidants; a highly nutritious vegetable.

COMMENTS: You will probably have to buy seeds only once. Purslane will self-sow.

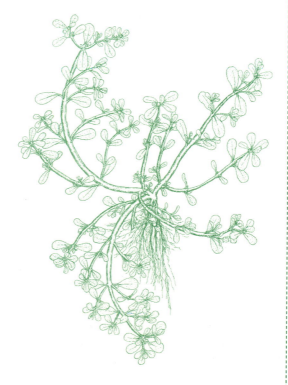

The very best green source of omega-3 fatty acids is free for the picking. It is purslane and there is probably some growing through a crack in your sidewalk now. This little wild green with its fleshy stems and spoon-shaped leaves grows just about everywhere in summer, but is easiest to spot in dry areas, where its exceptional drought resistance gives it an edge.

Wondrously rich in antioxidants, purslane contains the compound glutathione, an antioxidant and immune system stimulator. According to Dr. James Duke, purslane is the best plant source of vitamins A, C, and E. It is also rich in magnesium, which may prevent cluster headaches.

Look for wild purslane in early summer and try some, either in a salad or stir-fried. I find its taste delicious—a combination of nuttiness and citrus. If you like it, order seeds of purslane so that you'll have plenty to eat regularly.

Seed catalogs carry several varieties of purslane (see Sources). The advantage of growing your own from seed is that the varieties offered by seed companies have been selected—usually for size and habit, but also for color. Garden purslane is about four times the height and girth of the wild form, and it tends to be more upright, so the plants stay clean. Golden or French purslane is yellow. Cultivated strains also tend to be milder in flavor.

Purslane in the garden is a culinary gold mine. This versatile plant can be eaten raw or cooked. It stands alone as a green vegetable or mixes well with other ingredients. In soups, its mucilaginous leaves and stems, like okra, are a thickening agent. Its gently piquant flavor adds pep to salads and blends well with elephant garlic and shallots in stir-fries.

Purslane couldn't be easier to grow. Start seeds when the ground has warmed up a bit in late spring, when there is no longer any danger of frost. It isn't fussy about soil and, once established, thrives with little care and no watering. In fact, you could seed it into cracks in the garden path. Its tolerance for drought makes it an excellent subject for containers (where its tendency to self-sow is less of a problem).

Harvest the leaves before the flowers appear. This will keep tender new growth coming. If you continue to do this, you'll have a steady source of greens until frost.

Stir-Fry Soup

Stir-frying the vegetables separately keeps them crunchy. You spoon them into bowls and pour the spicy chicken broth over them. I created this recipe to enjoy crisp vegetables in a soup.

    4 cups chicken broth, or 2 cans
    ¼ teaspoon hot pepper flakes (or more, to taste)
    1 teaspoon grated ginger
  1–2 large cloves garlic, thinly sliced
  1–2 lemongrass stalks, thinly sliced
      Some or all of the following (quantities are suggestions):
      Carrot, sliced into matchsticks (¼ cup)
      Shiitake mushrooms, stems removed, caps sliced in strips
      (½ cup)
      Snow peas (½ cup)
      Lamb's-quarters or spinach greens, cut in shreds (1 cup)
      Purslane, washed, drained, with thick stems removed (1 cup)
      Green onions, sliced into rounds (¼ cup)
      Soy sauce

1. Combine the chicken broth with the hot pepper flakes, ginger, garlic, and lemongrass in a saucepan. Bring to a simmer, then turn to low heat.
2. Begin stir-frying with the vegetables that take the longest time to cook. For example, start with carrot sticks; after a minute or two, add the shiitakes. Stir-fry for a minute before adding the snow peas, the lamb's-quarters, and, almost at the end, the purslane. Stir-fry until the purslane is a deep, grass green. Finally, add the green onion slices.
3. Spoon the vegetables into four bowls.
4. Strain the chicken broth through a sieve and pour over the vegetables. Season with soy sauce to taste and serve immediately.

YIELD: 4 servings

Rose

ROSA

BOTANICAL NAME: *Rosa* spp. and hybrids, Rosaceae.

COMMON NAME: Rose.

DESCRIPTION: Shrub.

Height: From 1 to 30+ feet.

Flowers: Variable; petals are edible.

Leaves: Often borne on thorny branches.

HARVEST: Hips when they form; petals anytime.

CULTURE: Variable, but usually in sun, rich soil, good drainage, and even moisture.

USE: Rose hips and seeds are the medicinal parts of the rose plant. Mentioned in the German Commission E's monographs, a tea made from an infusion of the hips and seeds is useful in healing inflammation of oral and pharyngeal mucosa. Petals are edible and may be used in potpourris; the hips are an excellent source of vitamin C in teas, sauces, soups.

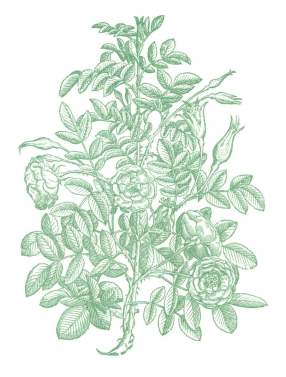

COMMENTS: Choose easy-care roses that need no chemicals.

$\mathcal{R}$oses need no introduction. They are easily the best-known and best-loved flower in the world. What many people don't know about roses is that their seedpods, or "hips," are incredibly nutritious. Some are estimated to be sixty times richer in vitamin C than oranges. When citrus fruits were scarce in Britain during World War II, hips from the wild dog rose *(Rosa canina)* were gathered by Girl and Boy Scouts to provide vitamin C for both civilian and military consumption.

Even with the free labor, it took a war for people to make use of the nutritionally rich bounty of wild roses. While rose petals for culinary use are easily harvested, gathering hips and then preparing them for use is labor intensive. Once you have a pound or two of hips, you have to deal with the seeds.

The classic method of dealing with rose hips involves stewing them and passing them through a food mill to remove the seeds and leathery skins. This produces a purée that is easy to work with, but doing so is not easy going and greatly reduces the end product. If you split the hips and remove as many seeds as possible as you go, or if you buy split rose hips with very few seeds, you can omit the food mill step, greatly decreasing kitchen mess and increasing the amount of stewed rose hips with which to cook.

Not all roses produce hips. Generally speaking, the single roses (those with a single row of petals around the center) and the semidouble roses are more likely to be pollinated—the first step toward forming hips. Densely petaled blooms, including many hybrid teas and centifolias, are less likely to form hips. And of course any rose that is cut will never bear fruit.

Noted for their hips are the species roses (naturally occurring roses that have not been hybridized) and rugosa roses, including some rugosa hybrids. The list below includes roses that are as lovely to look at as they are prolific in fruit.

BEAUTIFUL ROSES WITH BOUNTIFUL HIPS

R. 'Ballerina'   A 2- to 4-foot hybrid musk rose bearing hundreds of small pink flowers in clusters.

R. 'Blanc Double de Coubert'   A 4- to 6-foot hybrid rugosa rose with fragrant, semidouble white flowers.

R. 'Bonica'   An easy-care, 4-foot shrub rose with large clusters of many-petaled pink blooms.

R. 'Carefree Beauty'   An easy-care, 5-foot shrub rose; pink flowered, excellent for hedges.

R. 'Complicata'   An 8-foot shrub with deep pink single flowers with a white eye; can be trained as a climber.

R. 'Dortmund'   An easy-care hedger or climber with cherry-red, scented blooms.

R. 'Heritage'   A David Austin pink with delicious hips.

R. 'Old Blush'   A 4-foot China rose with fragrant blushed pink blooms.

Sweetbrier or Eglantine (R. eglanteria)   An 8- to 10-foot species rose with fragrant, bright pink, single blooms.

R. glauca   A 6-foot species rose with white-eyed, single pink flowers and darkly attractive foliage.

Swamp Rose (R. palustris)   A 6-foot native American species with dark pink flowers that tolerates heat and poorly drained sites.

If you start sampling rose hips off the bush (from organically grown roses, please!), you'll find that they vary in taste, size, and number of seeds. Some hips taste too sour, others may be too full of seeds. While the seeds are nutritious, they are too big to swallow easily. Making a purée is the first step toward using rose hips in a variety of dishes.

If you can remove enough seeds, you may not have to put the pulp through a food mill, a process I have found most unpleasant, uneconomical, and messy.

Preparing Rose Hip Purée

1. Gather rose hips. Wash them and allow them to dry. Snip off both ends of each hip with a scissors. Remove as many seeds as possible.
2. Place the hips in an enameled, stainless steel, or glass saucepan with about 2 cups of water for every pound of hips.
3. Cover and stew the hips for about 20 minutes.
4. Cool slightly and press through a sieve or food mill. If you have removed most of the seeds, this step is, happily, not necessary.

NOTE: The reddish brown purée may be frozen.

Rose Hip Coffee Cake

A yummy way to ingest vitamin C, this recipe uses whole rose hips from which the seeds have been removed. If you prefer to use rose hip purée that has been cooked, omit step 1. This recipe comes from Terry Pogue, whose radio show, Plant Talk, *was a favorite for listeners in the Washington, D.C., area. Since her retirement, Terry has become a computer whiz. She was always a fabulous cook.*

   1 cup rose hips, with seeds removed
   ½ cup sugar
   ¼ cup water
1½ cups flour
   ½ cup sugar
   ½ teaspoon baking powder
   ¼ teaspoon baking soda
   ¼ teaspoon salt
   ¼ cup butter, softened
   ½ cup plain yogurt
   1 egg
   1 teaspoon plus ¼ teaspoon vanilla
   2 tablespoons sliced almonds
   ⅓ cup powdered sugar
   2 teaspoons milk

1. Preheat the oven to 350°.
2. Combine the rose hips, sugar, and water in a small pot and bring to a boil. Turn down the heat and simmer, covered, for 5 to 10 minutes, or until the leathery hips turn tender. Remove the cover and reduce the mixture to a jam-like consistency. Cool.
3. In a large bowl, mix the flour, sugar, baking powder, baking soda, and salt.
4. Cut in the butter, mixing until the batter is evenly granular.
5. In another bowl, mix together the yogurt, egg, and 1 teaspoon of the vanilla. Add this mixture to the dry mixture and stir until blended.
6. Spoon two-thirds of the batter into a greased and floured 10-inch tube pan.

7. Spoon the rose hip mixture over the batter in the pan. Cover with the remaining batter. Top with the sliced almonds.
8. Bake for 35 to 45 minutes. Prick to see if a fork comes out clean.
9. Mix the powdered sugar, milk, and ¼ teaspoon vanilla and drizzle over the top of the warm cake.

YIELD: 6 to 8 servings

Cold Season Rose Hip Chili

Rose hips are traditionally made into jams and jellies. Their powerhouse of nutrients deserves inclusion in serious food. I reasoned that rose hips, like tomatoes, have an enticing sweet-sour flavor that lends itself well to chili. Loaded with vitamin C, rose hip chili arms the body and warms the soul.

  2 cups rose hips, seeds removed (as many as is humanly possible)
  3 cups beef bouillon
  3 tablespoons olive oil
  1 onion, chopped
  1 clove garlic, chopped
  ½ pound ground round
  1 tablespoon chili powder
2–3 dried chilis (the heat is up to you)
  1 teaspoon cinnamon
  1 teaspoon salt (or to taste)
  2 cups cooked kidney or black beans, or 1 can (washed and drained) beans

1. Microwave the rose hips in one cup of the bouillon for about 5 minutes at low power, or until soft. Set aside.
2. Heat the oil in a saucepan and add the onion and garlic. Cook until soft, about 5 minutes.
3. Add the ground round. Cook until the meat is brown. Pour off the fat.
4. Add the rose hips, the remaining bouillon, and the chili powder, chili

peppers, cinnamon, and ¼ teaspoon of the salt. Cook, covered, for 30 minutes.

5. Add the beans. Cook 15 minutes. Add salt to taste.

YIELD: 4 to 6 servings

The Only Good Fruitcake

This recipe for fruitcake is an adaptation of a recipe I clipped from a magazine twenty-seven years ago. Over the years, I've modified it. One change, the addition of rose hips and dried fruits and nuts to this cake's batter in place of the originally specified candied fruit, makes an enormous difference. By the way, the batter is intoxicating.

      2 cups sugar
   1½ cups butter, softened
      6 eggs
      ¼ cup molasses
      4 cups all-purpose flour
   2½ teaspoons baking powder
      2 teaspoons ground nutmeg
      1 cup rose hips, seeds carefully removed
      1 cup dried cherries
      1 cup dried pineapple, diced
      1 cup marmalade
      1 cup sunflower seeds
      5 cups pecans
      1 cup Kentucky bourbon plus additional for soaking cheesecloth
        wrapper

1. Preheat the oven to 250°.
2. Cream the sugar and butter until pale lemon color. Add the eggs, beating after each one.
3. Add the molasses. Mix well.
4. In another bowl combine the flour, baking powder, and nutmeg.

5. In a third bowl, combine the fruits, marmalade, sunflower seeds, and pecans. Add one cup of the flour mixture to coat the fruit.

6. Add the remainder of the flour mixture, alternating with the bourbon, to the creamed sugar and butter. Mix well.

7. Stir in the fruit mixture.

8. Grease one 10-inch tube pan or two 9×5×3-inch loaf pans. Line with greased brown paper.

9. Spoon the batter into the pan(s); cover with greased brown paper. (I use a stick of butter like a crayon on pieces of brown paper shopping bags, cut to size.)

10. Bake 2½ to 3 hours.

11. When cake is cool, remove the paper and wrap the cake in cheesecloth or muslin that has been soaked in bourbon. Wrap tightly in foil and store until ready to use.

YIELD: 20 servings

Joan's Mast-O-Khiar

This lovely Persian salad combines cucumbers and herbs. Dried, crumbled rose petals are an exotic and beautiful garnish.

1 English cucumber, peeled, diced, salted, and drained
16-ounce container of plain yogurt
¼ cup chopped green onions
2 cloves garlic, crushed
1 tablespoon chopped fresh mint
2 tablespoons chopped fresh dill
Salt and pepper
Dried rose petals (see note)

1. Mix the cucumber with the yogurt, green onions, garlic, mint, and dill. Season with salt and pepper.

2. Garnish with crumbled rose petals.

NOTE: Dry rose petals on an upturned basket, several days ahead.

YIELD: 4 servings

Rose Water

Make rose water as you would sun tea.

1. Gather fresh, scented flowers that have not been sprayed or treated with chemicals (including systemics).
2. Check for bugs before placing the whole flowers in a clean pint or quart jar.
3. Cover with hot water and let the jar sit in the sun for a day or two.
4. Strain and bottle the rose water. Refrigerate. Use as a hair rinse, or instead of water for lemonade.

Rosemary

ROSMARINUS OFFICINALIS

BOTANICAL NAME: *Rosmarinus officinalis,* Lamiaceae.

COMMON NAME: Rosemary.

DESCRIPTION: Tender perennial subshrub.

> *Height:* To 8 feet.

> *Flowers:* Blue.

> *Leaves:* Highly aromatic, thin, leathery; edible.

HARVEST: As needed.

CULTURE: Zones 8 to 10; sun; well-drained, neutral soil.

USE: May help prevent the breakdown of acetylcholine in the brain. A culinary herb.

COMMENTS: Like bay, rosemary requires good drainage but will die if allowed to dry out. 'Arp' is a hardy cultivar, supposedly to Zone 6.

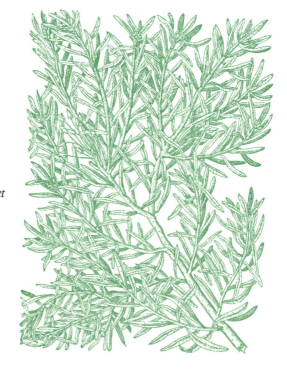

There's rosemary, that's for remembrance; pray you, love, remember.
—Shakespeare, *Hamlet*

$\mathcal{R}$osemary is yet another herb whose reputation in folk wisdom is now enjoying scientific validation. Since ancient times, rosemary has been the herb associated with both memory and remembrance. It is said that Greek scholars wore garlands of rosemary to quicken memory.

It is quite possible that these garlands did the trick. According to Dr. James Duke, rosemary's compounds, which can be absorbed through the skin, prevent the breakdown of acetylcholine. Rosemary may be useful in the prevention and treatment of Alzheimer's disease. In animal studies, it reduces the incidence of cancer.

The German Commission E lists infusions of cut rosemary leaves as approved for dyspepsia, rheumatic diseases, and circulatory problems.

Rosemary is easy to locate and grow. Though it is hardy only to very protected parts of Zone 7, it does well in a container inside over the winter. There is a cultivar of rosemary, 'Arp,' that is winter hardy to the Washington, D.C., area, where I live. Even so, I have lost several plants of 'Arp' that have been left outside all winter. This may have more to do with cold, wet clay soil than with absolute temperature. Make sure your soil drains fast. A good additive for clay soil is chicken grit.

Even with the chicken grit–enriched soil, I dig my rosemary up in fall, at about the time of the first frost. It is always surprising how gracefully rosemary tolerates being transplanted out of the garden and into a pot. After potting it, I move it into shade, close to where it had grown all summer, in order to let it get used to reduced light gradually.

Having it indoors means snippets of rosemary are always at hand. Even if rosemary had no medicinal value, it would be a culinary necessity. Imagine roast lamb or pork without it. It is superb in rosemary butter—melted over shredded carrots or baked sweet potatoes. It lends a unique flavor to a glass of after-dinner port and is terrific in baked goods such as scones, bread, and shortbread.

> **TIP**
>
> - *Enhance your port or other wines by inserting a sprig of rosemary in the bottle.*
> - *Place a sprig in your shampoo bottle.*
> - *Sprinkle rosemary leaves in your bath.*

Rosemary Shortbread

Sometimes only something very rich does the trick. Try a slice of this shortbread with a cup of tea on a dark, rainy winter afternoon. This was served several years ago at a garden club meeting at which I was speaking. I am sorry not to remember the club, the date, or the name of the member whose recipe it was. I remember only the ingredients she tossed off and how delicious the shortbread was.

⅓ cup sugar
1¼ cups flour
½ teaspoon salt
½ teaspoon baking soda
¼ pound unsalted butter
½ teaspoon finely chopped rosemary

1. Preheat the oven to 350°.
2. Mix together the dry ingredients.
3. Microwave the butter (on low) with the rosemary until the butter is melted.
4. Pour the butter mixture over the dry ingredients and mix until blended.
5. Roll out into an 8- to 10-inch circle and place it in a nonstick spring-form pan. (Or you can press the dough in with your fingers; in that case, the surface won't be smooth.)
6. Prick the dough with a fork.
7. Bake for 20 to 25 minutes, or until the shortbread is lightly browned on the edges.
8. Cut into wedges while still hot.

YIELD: 8 servings

Mary Cooper's Rosemary Cookies

Mary Cooper doesn't know this, but callers at her big, old house on the Mississippi in New Orleans scheme to time their visits in the hope that she will offer coffee and her famous rosemary cookies.

½ cup soft butter
½ cup confectioner's sugar
1 cup unbleached flour
1 tablespoon fresh rosemary leaves, finely chopped
Granulated sugar for stamping

1. Preheat the oven to 350°.
2. Cream the butter and sugar, then add the flour and rosemary.
3. On cookie sheets, spoon small teaspoonfuls of dough, about 3 inches apart.
4. Press with the bottom of a glass or a cookie press, dipped in sugar.
5. Bake for 10 to 12 minutes, or until brown. Cool and store in an airtight container.

YIELD: 30 to 36 cookies

Saffron

CROCUS SATIVUS

BOTANICAL NAME: *Crocus sativus,* Iridaceae.

COMMON NAMES: Saffron, autumn crocus.

DESCRIPTION: Perennial bulb.

> *Height:* To 8 inches.

> *Flowers:* Lavender, with edible, scarlet stamens in fall.

> *Leaves:* Narrow, from the base.

HARVEST: As soon as flowers open, remove the three scarlet stigmas from each.

CULTURE: Zones 6 to 9, sun to part shade in well-drained soil.

USE: Blood purifier, blood pressure reducer, nerve tonic, culinary spice.

COMMENTS: It is very easy to miss the fall flowering unless you inspect your plants daily.

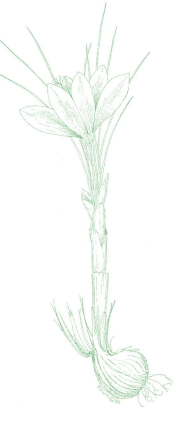

You've probably heard or read statements about saffron—estimates of how many thousands of flowers are required to compose a pound—that make it seem futile to attempt to grow it. True, it's expensive, but a pound of saffron is a lot of saffron and hundreds of times more than most people would use in a very long time.

Saffron is composed of the dried red stigmas of fall-blooming crocuses that grow from bulbs, and it really isn't hard to grow some for culinary use. All you have to do is buy the bulbs, complete little packages of embryonic life (see Sources), plant them two inches deep in a fairly sunny place with good drainage, and, presto, a soft lavender crocus emerges from each bulb in the fall. In subsequent years, the bulbs multiply, and unless you make a lot of paella, you will very soon have enough saffron to last you through the year.

If there is a problem with growing saffron, it is the harvest. You have to be there at the right time. This means checking your bulbs every single day in October and removing the three red stigmas from each flower as soon as it starts to open. I used to wait until the flowers opened completely because they are beautiful, especially with those elegantly draping stigmas. Trying to find just the right moment, after the flower faded but before the stigmas began to decompose, often meant missing the harvest.

My next strategy was to carefully remove the stigmas from the flowers as soon as they opened, but that left the blossoms looking ravaged. Now I am ruthless and harvest the whole flower. Part of the reason for ruthlessness is competition. Almost as soon as a flower opens, ants arrive and appear to eat the stigmas. They seem to be the only insects that actually eat them, but they are not the only ones drawn to the wonderfully seductive and intoxicating saffron flower. Frequently I have come upon a blooming saffron crocus and discovered, deep within the flower, what look like tiny drunken bees sleeping off a binge. Ladybugs, and other tiny insects, as well, appear oddly disoriented when I dislodge them.

Perhaps it is the crocetin, a chemical that lowers blood pressure in humans, in the saffron that has mellowed them. Or perhaps the saffron flower is a kind of insect spa. Natural healers use saffron as a nerve and heat tonic, a blood cleanser and a blood thinner. Saffron may also help relieve memory problems caused by circulatory disease.

Once I've dislodged the competition, I remove the three red stigmas from each flower and place them in a shallow bowl to dry. This takes a day or two and shrinks each stigma, or "thread," to perhaps half its original size—from about two inches to just under one inch long.

Using Saffron

To maximize saffron's rich color and flavor, steep it in boiling water. This recipe is for 1 teaspoon. Adjust according to the recipe you are using.

1. In a mortar, grind 1 teaspoon of saffron threads to a fine powder.
2. Add 2 tablespoons of boiling water. Stir.
3. Allow to cool before using.

Joan Aghevli's Saffron Ice Cream

Nothing on earth yields the color saffron but saffron. Mixed with rose water, saffron gives this ice cream a delightfully unusual taste. You can enrich the flavor by substituting half-and-half or whipping cream for the milk.

> 1 teaspoon saffron threads
> 4 egg yolks
> 1 teaspoon cornstarch
> ½ cup sugar
> 2 cups milk
> 2 teaspoons rose water (available at Middle Eastern grocery stores)

1. Grind the saffron using a mortar and pestle and soak in 2 tablespoons of boiling water. Allow to cool.
2. Combine the egg yolks, cornstarch, and sugar in a mixer bowl and beat until they are nearly white.
3. While they are beating, heat the milk to a boil, then ladle a cup or so into the egg mixture (with the beaters running).
4. Pour the contents of the mixing bowl, along with the saffron and the rose water, into the remaining heated milk. Cook over low heat until it thickens. *Do not boil* or the mixture will curdle. Remove from the heat. Cool in the refrigerator before using an ice-cream machine.
5. Taste. Add more rose water if desired.
6. Process in an ice-cream machine.

YIELD: 6 to 8 servings

Nora's Saffron Risotto
with Shrimp and Peas

Nora Pouillon of Restaurant Nora and Asia Nora in Washington, D.C., makes this delicious and comforting risotto.

    1 pound shrimp, peeled and deveined (if frozen, defrost under
       cold running water)
    2 tablespoons olive oil
    1 small onion, chopped
    2 cloves garlic, minced
1–1½ cups arborio rice, such as organic Cal Riso
    ¼ teaspoon saffron threads
    ½ cup white wine, optional
    3 cups chicken stock or water, heated to simmering
    1 cup frozen peas, defrosted
    ½ cup grated Parmesan, optional
       Salt and pepper
       Italian parsley or thyme for garnish

1. Sauté the shrimp in ½ tablespoon of the olive oil in a heavy sauté pan until they are pink. Remove from heat and set aside.
2. In the same pan, heat the remaining oil, add the onion, cook for 2 minutes until it is soft, then add the garlic and sauté 1 minute.
3. Add the rice and saffron, stirring until the rice grains are glistening. Then add the wine and 2 cups of the stock. Stir and cook until the liquid is almost absorbed, about 15 minutes.
4. Add the rest of the stock as you continue cooking and stirring, until the rice is creamy but still firm to the bite, about 20 minutes.
5. Add the shrimp, peas, and Parmesan. Taste, add salt and pepper if necessary, and heat through.
6. Serve garnished with fresh Italian parsley or a sprig of thyme.

NOTE: As a time-saver and a great convenience for entertaining, you can cook the rice ahead of time for 5 to 8 minutes, then cool. To finish, sauté the vegetables, fish, or meat of your choice, add the pre-cooked risotto and as much liquid (white wine, stock, or water) as necessary to cook the vegetables, and reheat the risotto. Stir to combine, bring to a boil, and cook until the risotto develops the consistency of creamy cereal.

YIELD: 4 servings

Sage

SALVIA OFFICINALIS

BOTANICAL NAME: *Salvia officinalis,* Lamiaceae.

COMMON NAME: Sage.

DESCRIPTION: Shrubby, evergreen perennial.

Height: To 30 inches.

Flowers: White or blue in spikes at the ends of branches in early summer.

Leaves: Aromatic, gray-green, crinkled leaves are edible; they have a taste that gets stronger if they are dried.

HARVEST: As needed; or cut small bunches to hang in the kitchen.

CULTURE: Zones 4 to 10. Sage grows well in full sun and requires excellent drainage; in warmer zones a mulch of gray or white stones may inhibit the fungus to which it is prone. Prune in spring to encourage a bushy habit. Sage discourages white cabbage moths in companion planting.

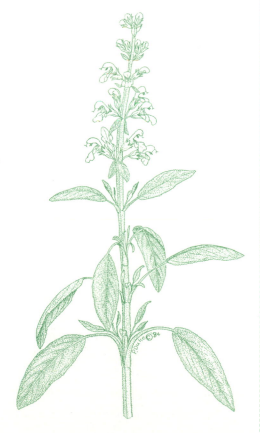

USE: Medicinally as a gargle or tea; in soups, dressings, stews, with poultry and meats.

COMMENTS: Excessive use of sage (far more than 3 cups of strong tea daily) may cause convulsions.

OTHER VARIETIES: Tricolored sage (*Salvia officinalis* 'Tricolor') is a pretty variegated mix of cream, green, and purple; purple sage (*S. officinalis* 'Purpurea') has purple-green leaves.

Eat sage in old age.
—Chinese proverb

Sage would be worth growing for its good looks alone. Its loosely spreading habit softens the edges of paths and cascades gracefully over walls. Softly colored gray-green leaves blend splendidly with other herbs, variegated foliage, and pastel flowers. The fact that sage is evergreen ensures an ever-ready supply of fresh leaves. You can run out to the garden on Thanksgiving morning and harvest fresh sage for turkey dressing.

Because of its strongly distinctive taste, sage is not as broadly used as herbs like thyme and parsley. Where its taste is appropriate, it is essential. Turkey dressing, sausages, pork, fish, duck, goose, and chicken soup all benefit from the flavor of sage.

Sage is an antiseptic. As a fungicide and antibacterial agent, it has been shown to inhibit organisms that resist penicillin—particularly in the treatment of sore throats and mouth sores. The German Commission E includes sage leaf on its approved list for treating inflammation of mucous membranes of the nose and mouth, as well as rating it effective for excessive perspiration. A gargle containing sage is definitely worth a try.

According to James Duke, sage, like rosemary, inhibits the enzyme that breaks down acetylcholine and may prevent or treat Alzheimer's disease. Once again, scientific research supports an ancient bit of folk wisdom: "In old age, eat sage."

Dr. Duke has also analyzed the nutrient content of sage tea, made with a teaspoon of the dried herb in a cup of boiled water. It contained more than the RDA (recommended daily allowance) of iron and magnesium and about half the RDA for calcium and potassium. It was also a significant source of zinc.

Sage Oatcakes

These oatcakes came about in an effort to re-create the oatcakes I was served in Scotland. That didn't happen. In fact, these are nothing like the originals. I like to think they are the kind of plain fare you might take with tea in a shepherd's hut in the lean, rugged Scottish Highlands. I've tried gussying them up with thyme, pepper, and crumbled bacon, but in the end I decided that their rustic simplicity is best. Delicious with honey for breakfast, they are also an unusual and nutritious accompaniment to a hearty winter soup.

 1 ounce butter
 ½ cup boiling water
 3 cups oatmeal
 1 tablespoon fresh sage, or ½ teaspoon dried
 ½ teaspoon baking soda
 1 teaspoon salt, approximately

1. Preheat the oven to 350°.
2. Melt the butter in the boiling water. Allow to cool.
3. Mix the oatmeal, sage, baking soda, and salt in a bowl.
4. Add the cooled liquid to the dry mix and stir to form a soft dough, adding more water if necessary (if the mixture doesn't stick together, the cakes won't).
5. Pat the dough into a round bottomless pan about 8 inches in diameter (a springform pan works well).
6. Place on an ungreased baking sheet and bake 40 minutes.
7. Cut into 8 wedges and let cool.

YIELD: 8 servings

SAGE GARGLE

Make a tea by pouring 1 cup of water that has just boiled over 2 teaspoons of the dried herb. Allow to steep for 10 minutes. Cool and use as a gargle.

Sage Applesauce

This applesauce isn't the cloying sweet stuff you get in cans. Sage gives it a deeper taste and enough character to stand up to wild game or roast lamb.

    6 tart apples, peeled, cored, and cut into ½-inch slices
    1 tablespoon sugar
      Pinch of salt
      Lemon juice, optional
    1 teaspoon finely chopped fresh sage

1. Put the apple slices into a microwavable bowl.
2. Sprinkle the slices with sugar and salt, or lemon juice, if the apples are not tart.
3. Add the sage. Mix all the ingredients together.
4. Cover the bowl and microwave on high for about 6 minutes, or until the apples are soft enough to mash.

YIELD: 6 servings

Saint-John's-wort

BOTANICAL NAME: *Hypericum perforatum,* Guttiferae.

COMMON NAMES: Saint-John's-wort, Klamath weed.

DESCRIPTION: Perennial.

Height: To 2 feet.

Flowers: Small, starry yellow flowers that bloom at midsummer, with red stamens that contain hypericin.

Leaves: Small, soft, light green, with tiny oil glands that look like perforations. Like the flowers, they are used in medicinal preparations.

HARVEST: In midsummer when the flowers are in bloom.

CULTURE: Sun to part shade; well-drained, ordinary soil.

USE: In teas and tinctures as an antidepressant, antianxiety remedy. The oil is helpful for burns, bruises, and cuts.

COMMENTS: Cattle that graze on large amounts of Saint-John's-wort exhibit sun sensitivity. It is thought to increase human sensitivity to sun and tendency to sunburn.

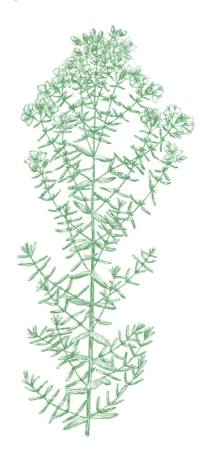

*E*ver since the German government set up its Commission E to investigate the medicinal properties of herbs, and approved Saint-John's-wort for depression, anxiety, and nervous unrest, this herb has been in the news. Saint-John's-wort's more than two-thousand-year history in folk medicine as an antidepressant has been vindicated. For mild depression and anxiety, Saint-John's-wort has been found to be just as effective as some pharmaceuticals but with fewer side effects (such as falls among elderly patients who take antidepressants).

In Germany alone, physicians write more than three million prescriptions a year for Saint-John's-wort. People suffering from severe, chronic depression, however, should consult a physician before trying this herb. Saint-John's-wort should not be taken with any other antidepressants.

This herb's fame as a mood lifter has almost eclipsed its other healing properties. There is a long tradition in folk medicine of using oil of St.-John's-wort to hasten the healing of burns, cuts, and bruises. Research has demonstrated that Saint-John's-wort does have antibacterial and antiviral properties. Exciting new studies are examining Saint-John's-wort's potent antiretroviral activity. The herb is currently being investigated for use with AIDS patients.

Very easy to grow, Saint-John's-wort is considered a weed in some areas. In the Pacific Northwest, it is called Klamath weed. Seeds are available (see Sources). You can either start plants indoors to transplant out or sow seeds outside where the plants are to grow. Select a well-drained place in sun or light shade. Saint-John's-wort isn't particular about soil fertility.

A rhizomatous perennial plant that develops woody stems, Saint-John's-wort grows about two feet tall, but tends to sprawl. Its delicate leaves and yellow, star-shaped flowers are attractive in the front of a border.

Harvest leaves and flowers just as the flowers open. Dry in an airy place and store for a soothing tea.

Saint-John's-wort Oil

Go the whole route and time your preparation of this oil for Midsummer Day. After the dew has dried, cut the leaves and flowers of Saint-John's-wort, leaving only about 6 inches on the plants. Making this healing red oil couldn't be easier. Rub it onto bruises or sunburned skin.

Saint-John's-wort tops and flowers
Virgin olive oil, to cover

1. Place the Saint-John's-wort tops (stems and leaves) and flowers in a jar that is large enough to hold them with some headroom.
2. Cover with the olive oil. Add an extra inch above the tops and flowers. Make sure they are completely covered with oil or they may spoil.
3. Cover the jar and place it in a sunny window. Shake vigorously every day.
4. Over 5 or 6 weeks, the oil will gradually turn red. When it is bright red, it is done.
5. Strain the oil through cheesecloth or a coffee filter, bottle it, and store the bottle in a cool, dark place. Use as needed. It will probably keep for three months.

Saw Palmetto

SERENOA REPENS

BOTANICAL NAME: *Serenoa repens,* Palmae.

COMMON NAMES: Saw palmetto, palmetto.

DESCRIPTION: Tender palm.

Height: To 12 feet.

Flowers: Small, fragrant, creamy white in summer, followed by medicinal berries that mature in early winter.

Leaves: Large, up to 3 feet across, palm fronds in blue- to yellow-green.

HARVEST: Fruits when they are ripe, in early winter.

CULTURE: Zones 9 to 10, sun to light shade, good drainage.

USE: Fruits, dried and made into teas, tinctures, decoctions.

COMMENTS: A handsome native palm.

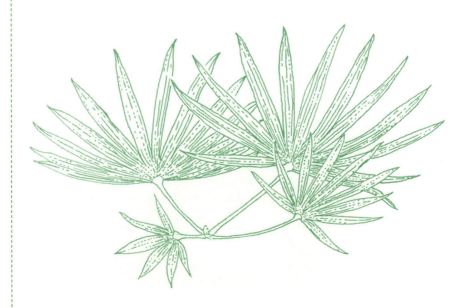

Saw palmettos are a common sight growing wild throughout Florida and in the coastal areas of South Carolina and Georgia. Native Americans and early settlers learned to value the blue-black fruits of the saw palmetto as a tonic for both people and animals. In folk medicine, saw palmetto fruits enjoyed the reputation of being an aphrodisiac.

While this reputation may or may not be deserved, saw palmetto has been used successfully to shrink enlarged prostates in men with mild BPH, or benign prostatic hyperplasia, stages 1 and 2, thus restoring more normal urinary function. It is on the German Commission E's approved list for this use and is considered a first-line treatment for BPH in Germany. Because BPH affects more than 50 percent of men over their lifetimes, and for its potential in preventing hair loss, saw palmetto is coming to be known as a men's herb.

This rise in popularity has caused problems in Florida, where harvesters, working for wholesale brokers who sell to the pharmaceutical industry, strip the berries from plants on public lands and private property, severely depriving wildlife. In an article titled "The Ethics of Wildcrafting," Linda Thornton writes: "Saw palmetto provides some form of sustenance to 100 bird species, 27 mammal species, 25 amphibians, 61 reptiles, and many insect species."

If you live in a warm climate where saw palmettos are hardy, you can grow them as handsome additions to your home landscaping. That way, you'll be able to grow enough berries to share with the birds and the beasts.

However, this is another herb that, for medicinal use, may be better purchased in standardized form. According to naturopathic physician Dr. Michael T. Murray, in the treatment of BPH, a fat-soluble standardized saw palmetto extract is more effective than the crude berries.

Still, some effect is better than none. And it's easy to make a tincture from the berries if you have them.

Prostate-Preserving Tonic

Use a coffee grinder to grind the berries.

    1 ounce saw palmetto berries, ground
    10 ounces (280 ml) 190 proof food-grade alcohol (available at
       liquor stores)

1. Put the ground berries into a jar.
2. Pour the alcohol over the berries. Cover and shake vigorously.
3. Shake once or twice a day for a month.
4. Pour the tincture through a coffee filter. Bottle and store in a cool
   place, out of the light. Brown or dark bottles are best.

Spinach

SPINACIA OLERACEA

BOTANICAL NAME: *Spinacia oleracea,* Cheropodiaceae.

COMMON NAME: Spinach.

DESCRIPTION: Annual.

Height: 8 to 10 inches.

Flowers: Cut before flowering.

Leaves: Edible, can be crinkled or smooth.

HARVEST: Cut plants at ground level when the leaves are 6 inches long.

CULTURE: Sun to very light shade in fertile, nearly neutral soil; thin plants to stand 6 to 8 inches apart.

USE: Compounds in spinach relax the heart muscle. A highly nutritious vegetable.

COMMENTS: Spinach grows best in cool weather.

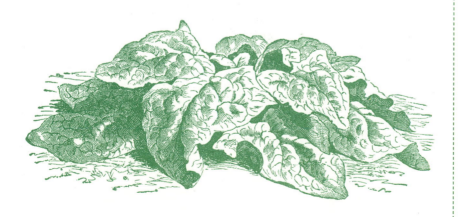

Cooked spinach was rated the second-healthiest vegetable (after collard greens) in a list published by the independent, nonprofit Center for Science in the Public Interest. Vegetables were rated by percentage of vitamins, minerals, and health-enhancing compounds they contained. The very best food source of zinc, generously endowed spinach also boasts antioxidant carotenoids, vitamin C, folate, postassim, calcium, magnesium (a half cup cooked contains 75 milligrams), iron, and fiber. Spinach also contains vitamin K, which plays a role in allowing proteins to be taken up by the bones, making them stronger.

While it is included here because it is nutritionally superb, spinach is indispensable in the kitchen. The most versatile of vegetables, it can be served raw in salads, stir-fried, steamed, or stewed.

Spinach is a cool-weather crop, started in early spring while there are still light frosts and again at the end of summer for a fall crop. It also grows over winter in a cold frame. Hot weather will cause spinach to bolt.

Thin spinach to stand 6 to 8 inches apart and eat the thinnings. Spinach leaves mature at about six inches long, but you can harvest it at any time you think it is big enough to be worth the effort.

Shiitake Creamed Spinach

I first tried the combination of spinach and shiitakes in one of François Dionot's classes at l'Academie de Cuisine. Since then, I've become a shiitake junkie, keeping dried ones in the pantry for times when the fresh were not at hand. A tiny bit of butter and cream give this combination of healing shiitakes and nutrient-rich spinach richness without adding too much fat.

    2 teaspoons butter
    ½ cup chopped shallots
    ½ cup shiitakes (about 5 or 6), with stems discarded, caps sliced
    2 supermarket bags of spinach leaves, washed and destemmed
        Salt and pepper
    2 tablespoons half-and-half
    1 teaspoon flour

½ cup bread crumbs, optional, for topping

1 tablespoon Parmesan, optional, for topping

1. Melt the butter in a saucepan. Add the shallots and cook 2 to 3 minutes.
2. Add the shiitakes. Cook 3 minutes.
3. Add the spinach, one-fourth at a time, salting and peppering lightly as you go. Cook until all of the spinach is wilted and dark green.
4. In a cup or small bowl, mix a few drops of the half-and-half with the flour to make a paste. Add the rest of the half-and-half. Mix well and add to the spinach. Heat through.
5. If you wish, spoon the spinach into a casserole and sprinkle bread crumbs and Parmesan over the top. Place in a 350° oven for 10 to 15 minutes.

YIELD: 8 servings

Spinach and Ham Strudel

Sue Watterson's Asparagus and Ham Strudel (page 11) was so good and I made it so many times, I tried this adaptation just for variety. It's a great brunch or luncheon dish. You might also substitute cubed, cooked chicken for the ham.

2 large shallots, finely chopped

½ cup plus 1 tablespoon olive oil

1 pound spinach, washed, drained, and chopped (4 to 5 cups)
   Salt and pepper

6 sheets of phyllo dough, thawed

1 egg white, lightly beaten

4 ounces Parmesan, grated

½ pound ham, thinly sliced

1. Place the chopped shallots with 2 tablespoons of the olive oil in a large saucepan. Sauté until soft.
2. Add the spinach to the shallots. Season lightly with salt and pepper. Cook very slowly, allowing the water clinging to the leaves to evaporate.

3. Preheat the oven to 375°.

4. Place one sheet of phyllo dough on a clean, flat work surface, long side toward you. Brush with olive oil.

5. Place a second phyllo sheet on top of the first; brush the surface of the second sheet with oil. Repeat until you have a stack of five sheets.

6. Lay the sixth phyllo sheet on top of the others; brush the surface of this last sheet with some of the beaten egg white.

7. Sprinkle the grated Parmesan over the last phyllo layer, leaving a 2-inch border of dough on each side.

8. Place slices of ham, overlapping slightly, on top of the cheese in a single layer. Spoon the spinach evenly over the surface (it probably will not make a continuous layer).

9. Starting with the long end of the phyllo nearest you, start rolling the stacked sheets of dough around the filling. Roll gently but firmly in jelly roll fashion, until the filling is completely wrapped and you have a stuffed tube of dough. This is your strudel.

10. Carefully place the strudel on a lightly greased or parchment-lined baking pan. Brush the outside surface of the strudel with the remaining egg white.

11. Bake for 20 to 25 minutes, or until crisp and browned. Let stand for 5 minutes before slicing.

YIELD: 4 to 6 servings

Stevia

STEVIA REBAUDIANA

BOTANICAL NAME: *Stevia rebaudiana,* Asteraceae.

COMMON NAMES: Stevia, South American honeyleaf plant.

DESCRIPTION: Tender woody perennial.

Height: In containers, about 2 inches.

Flowers: Small, frothy, white at the tips of the stems.

Leaves: Light green, intensely sweet.

HARVEST: Cut as needed or cut back the entire plant in early summer when the plant is in active growth; dry the leaves quickly.

CULTURE: Zones 9 to 10 (and possibly Zone 8). In colder areas, grow or transplant in containers and bring inside to a very sunny window over winter. Needs fast drainage.

USE: A noncaloric sweetener.

COMMENTS: It is hard to gauge the correct amount of water the plant needs. Too wet and it dies, especially indoors. Too dry and whiteflies arrive.

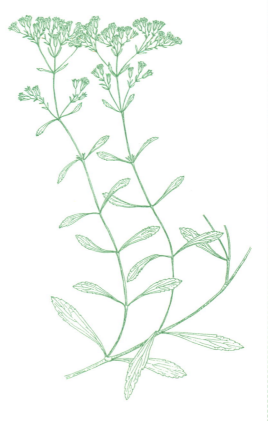

Currently . . . in North America, on average, each person eats 138 pounds of
sugar per year.   —Chanchal Cabrera, clinical herbalist, speaking
at the Fourth International Herb Symposium

$\mathcal{A}$dd sugar intake to inactivity and poor diet and it isn't any wonder that more than half the citizens of the United States are overweight. Being overweight brings on its own set of health problems. When excessive sugar in the diet is part of the picture, there is an additional threat: the consumption of large amounts of sugar depresses the immune system, leaving a person at greater risk of disease.

Having a sweet tooth as well as a violent allergic reaction to some artificial sweeteners, I found that stevia, a little plant from Paraguay, helped me wean myself from sugared teas. For centuries, stevia has safely sweetened food and drink in its native country. Now, the Japanese government has approved the use of stevia extract as a low-calorie sugar substitute in processed foods. In this country, stevia is sold labeled as a dietary supplement, not as a sweetener.

Experiments with concentrated steviosides (the compounds in stevia) indicate that they may impair fertility and promote heart and kidney failure.

Shortly after learning about stevia, I ordered plants by mail (see Sources). These were planted in the garden in places I fervently hoped approximated Paraguay: warm sites in full sun, in average soil with good drainage. As the plants showed a tendency to be lank, all three were cut back in June. They produced bushier growth as a result and made it through the summer. I was so sure they wouldn't make it through the Mid-Atlantic winter that I didn't even leave one plant outside to test hardiness. All three got transplanted into pots for the winter, but two died—as a result, I think, of rough transplanting.

The third has made it through winter in a pot in a west window, but not without incident. In January, the little stevia became infested with whitefly. In the frantic soapy baths and rinsing that ensued, several of stevia's rather brittle branches snapped off. Of these, one rooted (after being dipped in rooting hormone and placed in a moistened peat pellet) and has begun to produce new leaves. At the National Arboretum, cuttings from nonblooming stems of stevia plants are taken at a better time—mid-August.

If you want to use stevia as your main source of sweetener, two plants should suffice: a little stevia goes a long way. If you buy the powder, one teaspoon of finely ground leaves supposedly equals the sweetness of one cup of sugar. I find that one small, dried leaf or half of a large one crumbled in a cup of tea works for me. Or you can make stevia syrup and use it to add the precise amount of sweetness you prefer.

Stevia is not sugar. It has a different kind of sweetness. Before you invest in plants, buy a tincture of stevia from a health food store and try it. Or buy it in little packets—just like those of artificial sweeteners. Then, if you like it, buy a plant or two.

Stevia Syrup

Not thick like a true syrup, this recipe makes a stevia liquid that can be added to drinks.

　　2 tablespoons dried stevia leaves
　　1 cup boiling water

1. Rub the stevia leaves through a sieve.
2. Pour the boiling water over the leaves. Allow to cool. Strain.
3. Bottle the liquid, refrigerate, and use it to sweeten drinks.

Strawberry

FRAGARIA SPP.

BOTANICAL NAME: *Fragaria* spp., Rosaceae.

COMMON NAME: Strawberry.

DESCRIPTION: Perennial fruit.

> *Height:* To 12 inches.
>
> *Flowers:* Small; white petals around a yellow center.
>
> *Leaves:* Dark green, toothed; may be steeped for teas.

HARVEST: When ripe, usually early summer.

CULTURE: Zones 3 to 8; deep, rich soil with good drainage in sun. In the North, mulch to protect from cold. In the South, a mulch keeps the soil cool and the fruits clean.

USE: A highly nutritious food; leaf tea eases cramps and may help prevent cancer.

COMMENTS: Strawberry varieties perform differently in various climates. Consult your local agricultural extension agent for recommended types.

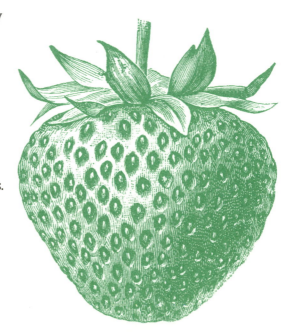

*A*ll berries are good for you, but strawberries consistently outrank other foods when rated nutritionally. In a list compiled by researchers at Tufts University, they were among the eleven best food sources of anti-oxidant compounds. "Healthy Foods," a booklet published by the non-profit Center for Science in the Public Interest, ranked strawberries third out of thirty-nine fruits for the percentage of U.S. RDA they provide.

Strawberries are especially rich in vitamin C. A half cup contains about 70 percent of the U.S. RDA for vitamin C. It also contains the mineral boron, which, according to Dr. James Duke, can boost the levels of estrogen circulating in the body—a boon for postmenopausal women. In Dr. Duke's database, strawberries are the top boron-containing food.

Versatile and delicious, strawberries are one of the easiest fruits to grow. Buy plants in late summer or early spring and set them into very fertile, moist soil. It is extremely important to get the crown—the disk from which the leaves emerge—at the right level. It should rest just at soil level, with all emerging growth above the soil and all roots below.

Strawberries send out runners to form new plants. Possibly because I grow strawberries in limited space, I find these confusing. I have neatened beds in autumn, allowing most of what was there to grow unchecked. Then, after two or three years, I simply ordered new plants and removed the strawberry bed to another part of the garden.

Delicious Alpine strawberries don't send out runners. Much smaller than regular strawberries, they can be grown very easily from seed and will produce a few of their tangy berries in their first year in the garden. They make great, well-behaved edgings or container plants.

Strawberries lend themselves to wonderful soups and delectable desserts. Strawberry leaf tea, rich in vitamins and minerals, also contains ellagic acid, touted as a cancer preventive. Like raspberry leaf tea, it may ease menstrual cramps by relaxing smooth muscle.

Strawberry Leaf Tea

1 cup boiling water (8 ounces)
½ cup fresh strawberry leaves (about 1 ounce)

1. Pour the boiling water over the fresh strawberry leaves.
2. Allow to steep for 15 to 20 minutes.

Sue's Strawberry Dessert Salad

Café Bethesda's talented chef Sue Watterson suggests serving this salad with al-mond biscotti or coconut ice cream—or both. To keep the strawberries firm, wait until the last minute to combine the ingredients.

> 1 quart strawberries
> Zest of 2 oranges
> ½ cup water
> ½ cup sugar
> ½ cup orange juice
> 1 teaspoon grated ginger
> Seeds of ½ vanilla bean
> ¼ cup orange-flavored liqueur (Triple Sec or Grand Marnier)
> 6–8 mint leaves, cut into fine threads

1. Wash and slice the strawberries. Set aside.
2. Julienne the orange zest, carefully omitting the bitter white part of the peel.
3. Cook the water, sugar, orange juice, ginger, and vanilla seeds into a syrup.
4. Add the orange zest to the hot syrup. Remove from the heat.
5. Allow the syrup to cool slightly. Add the liqueur.
6. Thread the mint.
7. To keep the strawberries firm, wait until shortly before serving to combine the strawberries, syrup, and finely threaded mint.

YIELD: 4 servings

Sumac

BOTANICAL NAME: *Rhus* spp., Anacardiaceae.

COMMON NAME: Sumac.

DESCRIPTION: Suckering tree.

> *Height:* To 15 feet.
>
> *Flowers:* Greenish white in summer.
>
> *Leaves:* Large compound leaves turn brilliant orange and red in fall.

HARVEST: Snap off the cones of berries as soon as they are deep red.

CULTURE: Zones 3 to 8. Beyond good drainage and sun, sumac requires little in the way of soil fertility or care; the colony-forming stems can be cut to the ground to control height.

USE: Roots were used in Native American medicine; the berries yield a tasty beverage that resembles pink lemonade.

COMMENTS: Poison sumac *(Rhus vernix)* has white berries.

SPECIES: There are beautiful, cut-leaf forms of the staghorn and smooth sumacs with the cultivar name 'Laciniata' that are great specimen trees for the home landscape.

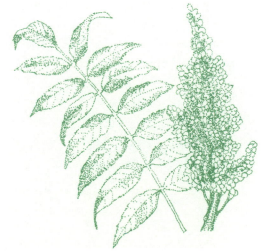

Sumacs are fast-growing trees that pop up along roadsides all over the country. We notice them in fall when their leaves turn scarlet and they bear red clusters of berries at the tips of the branches. There is also a poison sumac, but it is easy to distinguish because it has white berries. The red berries from the staghorn sumac *(Rhus typhina)*, the shining sumac *(Rhus copallina)*, and the smooth sumac *(Rhus glabra)* are all safe. The berries of a Mediterranean species *(Rhus coriaria)* yield "sumac," a condiment in Middle Eastern dishes.

Sumac berries grow in pointed, oblong clusters on female plants. It's easy (if you can reach them) to snap off the whole clusters from the ends of branches. Do this as soon as possible in late summer and early fall while they are still red.

Native Americans used the berries for cough syrups and to stop bed-wetting and cure mouth sores.

Sumac Drink and Sorbet

Both sumac-ade and sumac sorbet are a lovely watermelon pink. Their taste is gentle, a cross between lemonade and watermelon.

1. Gather sumac heads, rinse briefly, and pull the berries from the stems. Allow the berries to dry thoroughly.
2. Grind the berries in a coffee grinder.
3. Use 2 tablespoons ground berries to 8 ounces boiling water. Allow to steep as it cools.
4. Strain and sweeten to taste.

TO MAKE A SORBET:

5. Add ¼ cup sugar syrup to a cup of sumac juice and test for sweetness. Adjust to taste.
6. Put sumac juice into an ice-cream maker and follow manufacturer's directions.

Sunflower

BOTANICAL NAME: *Helianthus annuus,* Asteraceae.

COMMON NAME: Sunflower.

DESCRIPTION: Annual.

> *Height:* To 8 feet.

> *Flowers:* Yellow or white petals around a central disk of seeds.

> *Leaves:* Hairy, green.

HARVEST: Quickly, before the birds get the seeds, as soon as the petals dry.

CULTURE: Full sun; deep, rich soil.

USE: Nutritionally rich; may prevent prostate problems.

COMMENTS: Tall sunflowers may need staking.

OTHER SPECIES: Jerusalem artichoke *(Helianthus tuberosus),* a perennial with edible, tuberous roots.

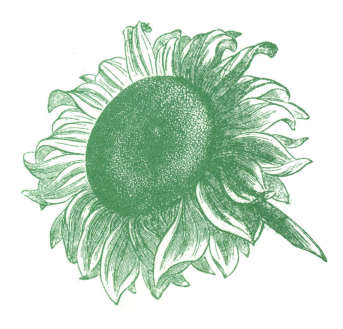

$\mathcal{M}$ost people are familiar with tall annual sunflowers. They are easy to grow, and they form a pretty background to a summer border. Varieties such as 'Russian Mammoth' and 'Giganteus' bear enormous flowers on plants that stand nine to fourteen feet high. Often a foot across, the flowers have petals set in rows around a large, central disk of cunningly arranged, edible seeds.

Generally speaking, gray or white sunflower seeds are considered eating seeds, or confectionery seeds, and the black ones are for pressing oil and use as birdseed. But the birds don't know this and will go after sunflower seeds of any color. It's hard to beat them to a flower head. Only once or twice have I managed to cut off a head before some busy bird has pecked away a few of the seeds, but I don't begrudge them a few of these nutritious seeds.

Birds have no problem getting through the tough outer shell of sunflower seeds, but people do. In *Feasting Free on Wild Edibles*, Bradford Angier suggests cracking the seeds first by rolling over them with a rolling pin, then putting them in a bowl of water. The shells will float and the heart meat sink to the bottom. This method works, but it takes some practice to arrive at just the right amount of pressure to crack the shells enough to free the meat without crushing it.

Rich in vitamin E, sunflower seeds also contain fatty acids, essential amino acids, and beta-carotene. Used in folk medicine in expectorant mixtures, they are currently being investigated for their role in the prevention of prostate gland problems.

Curing Sunflower Seeds

The Territorial Seed Company (see Sources) offers the following advice for curing sunflower seeds:

1. Use a gray-seeded variety like 'Giganteus.'
2. Cut the heads off after they begin to wither, and hang them upside down in a dry location away from rodents and birds.
3. Once the heads are dry, rub the seeds off and soak overnight in 1 gallon of water with 1 cup of salt added.
4. Dry in a 250° oven for 4 to 5 hours and store in an airtight container.

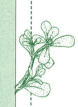

JERUSALEM ARTICHOKES

Perennial sunflowers have much smaller flowers and correspondingly smaller seeds than annual sunflowers. One, *Helianthus tuberosus,* the Jerusalem artichoke, makes up for its lack of edible seeds by producing edible roots, knobby tubers attached to thin roots that radiate out from the plant under the ground. For the best flavor, wait until after a hard frost to dig them. Scrub, dry, and store them in the refrigerator in a plastic bag. They keep for months.

A staple in the diet of Native Americans, Jerusalem artichokes, or sunchokes, contain vitamin A, thiamin, riboflavin, and only seven calories to half a cup when fresh. Don't peel off the flavorful skin, but do soak slices in lemon juice or salad dressing to keep them from discoloring. They add a lovely crunch to salads and stand in for water chestnuts in stir-fries.

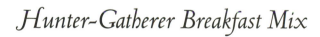

Hunter-Gatherer Breakfast Mix

Anthropologists examining ancient remains have found evidence of better health in the skeletons of hunter-gatherer people who subsisted on nuts, grains, berries, and whatever they could hunt than in those of later, "more advanced" agricultural civilizations. I think of this each time I prepare this mixture.

The hunter-gatherer mix is basically a custom assortment of dried fruits, seeds, and nuts to be sprinkled liberally over cereal. The kind you make yourself is always superior to cereals that you buy complete with fruits and nuts that never seem to contain enough of the "good stuff." They are expensive to boot. Having it on hand, ready mixed and convenient, will give you just the nutrients without the fuss on busy mornings. Custom-design a mix of sunflower seeds, nuts, dried fruit, and soybeans to add antiaging vitamin E and the mineral selenium, as well as fiber and monounsaturated fatty acids.

On calm days, I slice fruit into the bottom of a cereal bowl, top it with a fortified cereal, then add this delicious mix of nuts and dried berries. On wildly rushed days, the mix goes into a plastic bag with some crunchy cereal to be munched like trail mix in the car—not a particularly healthful practice, but better than a hasty doughnut and coffee or no breakfast at all.

SELECT AS MANY AS DESIRED FROM THE FOLLOWING:
   4 ounces sunflower seeds (contain vitamin E)
   1 cup wheat germ (aphrodisiac, general tonic)
   ½ cup ground flaxseed (omega-3 fatty acids, fiber)
   20 brazil nuts, chopped (very high in antioxidant selenium)
   4 ounces dried cherries (delicious, nutritious)
   4 ounces dried cranberries (help maintain a healthy urinary tract)
   4 ounces dried blueberries (great for your eyes)
   4 ounces almonds (contain vitamin E)
   4 ounces soy buds (processed soybeans; contain phytoestrogens)
   4 ounces pumpkin seeds (good for prostate)

1. Mix together the desired ingredients from the list above and store with a scoop in a covered canister.
2. Sprinkle the mix over fortified cereal or yogurt and chopped fruit for a crunchy and nutritious breakfast. Or, if you must, scoop into a plastic bag or recycled yogurt container, dash out the door, and munch en route to work.

Thyme

BOTANICAL NAME: *Thymus* spp., Labiatae.

COMMON NAMES: Thyme, lemon thyme.

DESCRIPTION: Evergreen subshrub.

> *Height:* To 2 feet.

> *Flowers:* Pink, lilac, or white.

> *Leaves:* The small, densely clustered leaves are edible and highly aromatic.

HARVEST: Pick thyme sprigs fresh as needed. The leaves are easier to strip off the tiny twigs when they are somewhat dry.

CULTURE: Grow thyme in full sun in well-drained soil.

USE: The antiseptic leaves flavor soups, stews, dressings.

COMMENTS: Thyme adapts well to container culture.

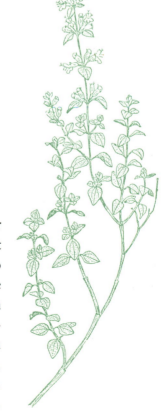

I would never be without fresh thyme for use in the kitchen, so it's great to know that an herb that adds such delectable flavor to foods also has medicinal properties. The German Commission E includes thyme on its approved list as an herbal remedy for upper respiratory catarrh. All thymes contain thymol, a powerful antiseptic. Knowing this, I use it freely in just about anything—soups, stews, salads, custards, dressings, stuffings.

Some people use the dried leaves for a tea that is reputed to help with hangovers.

In growing thyme, one factor that cannot be ignored is good drainage. In my garden, this more than the amount of sunlight has been crucial to the success of several species of thyme. Creeping thyme *(Thymus serpyllum)* thrives in a rock garden in bright light, but not full sun. Common thyme *(T. vulgaris)* and lemon thyme *(T. × citriodorus)* grow on a slope in clay soil that has been lightened with ample amounts of chicken grit. Thyme's need for drainage makes it an excellent subject for containers.

Thymes are actually subshrubs that become woody with age. When they begin to die back in the center, it's best to start anew. You can grow thyme from cuttings, taken in spring. Or you can buy new plants—a good opportunity to try different types. There is a broad-leaved thyme *(T. pulegioides)*, a caraway thyme *(T. herba-barona)*, and a woolly thyme *(T. pseudolanuginosus)*.

Of all the thymes, my favorite is lemon thyme because of its citrusy scent. It lends to chicken and beef dishes a rather exotic flavor that reminds me of Middle Eastern dishes. Lemon thyme is also wonderful thrown into the bath or cut into potpourri.

Homemade Zahtar

This recipe is my own variation on zahtar, a savory mix of seeds and spices from the Middle East. After you dip your bread into the olive oil, you coat it with a delectable mix of seeds and spices. Then you toast it. The classic recipe, given to me by Linda Sharif, combines two parts thyme to one part sumac and one part sesame seeds. This one is a bit different. Try either one for breakfast, toasted on a bagel.

    1½ teaspoons sumac powder (available in Middle Eastern
        groceries)
    2 teaspoons freshly dried thyme, crushed
    1 teaspoon sesame seeds
    1 teaspoon caraway seeds
    1 teaspoon of any other freshly dried, crumbled herb, optional
        Bagel
        Olive oil

1. Mix together the sumac and the seasonings and spread evenly on a shallow plate.
2. Dip a bagel into olive oil and then into the zahtar.
3. Toast in a toaster oven.

YIELD: 6 servings

Thyme-Ginger Dressing

An assertive combination that goes well with end-of-the-season lettuce.

1 teaspoon chopped thyme
1 teaspoon grated ginger
½ cup olive oil
1 tablespoon white wine vinegar
2 teaspoons white wine
    Pinch of sugar

1. Whisk all the ingredients together.
2. Drizzle over salad greens.

YIELD: 1 cup

Tomato

BOTANICAL NAME: *Lycopersicon lycopersicum,* Solanaceae.

COMMON NAME: Tomato.

DESCRIPTION: Annual fruit.

Height: To 5 feet.

Flowers: Small, yellow flowers are followed by large, usually red fruits.

Leaves: Deeply cut, on lax stems that need support.

HARVEST: The fruits when ripe.

CULTURE: Rich, moist soil in full sun.

USE: Tomatoes contain compounds, antioxidants that lower blood pressure, maintain prostate, and may fight cancer. The fruit is highly prized.

COMMENTS: No garden should be without them.

*T*omatoes are so essential and delicious a part of our diet that we would eat them even if they were not good for us. What serendipity that

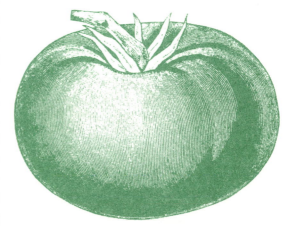

they are nutritional gold mines. In addition to potassium, ample vitamin C, and iron (best absorbed in the presence of vitamin C), they contain lycopene, a potent antioxidant carotenoid. Some researchers think lycopene may be twice as effective at fighting cancer as better-studied beta-carotene. Tomato's compounds also lower blood pressure and keep the prostate gland healthy. And, according to Dr. James Duke, tomatoes help to curb the symptoms of allergic conditions such as asthma because they are rich in vitamin C and contain flavonoids that inhibit the release of histamine.

Tomatoes are easy to grow if you can provide the one thing they absolutely require: sunshine. Buy plants, available at most garden centers, in midspring when it is safe to put these exceedingly frost-tender plants in the ground. It is also easy to grow them from seed in a sunny window, especially if you use peat pellets.

In addition to full sun, tomatoes, which are heavy feeders, need rich soil and ample, even moisture. Given these things, tomatoes produce heavily from about the Fourth of July until frost.

When the weatherman warns of the first fall frost, be sure to pick your tomatoes—both red and green—and bring them inside. Some people take in the entire plant and hang it up inside to let the tomatoes continue to ripen. If most of your tomatoes are green at this juncture, use any that are bruised or blemished for fried green tomatoes and store the rest. Tomatoes will continue to ripen indoors. Some have been especially bred for inside ripening. 'Longkeeper' is one that matures slowly, thus extending your enjoyment of homegrown tomatoes.

Fried Green Tomatoes à la Steve Durough

Steve is a great cook in the Southern tradition. He lives in Wilsonville, Alabama.

  3–4 green tomatoes
      Salt
      Pepper
  1 cup flour
      Vegetable oil

1. Slice the green tomatoes ⅓-inch thick. Lay them out on a china plate (you can add a second layer). Salt heavily and leave about 1 hour.
2. Pour off the watery juice but do not rinse the tomato slices.

3. Pepper the tomato slices, dip them in flour, and fry in ¼ inch of vegetable oil about 5 minutes on each side. The outsides should be crispy and brown and the insides soft.

YIELD: 6 to 8 servings

X's Aunt's Tomato Chutney

The following recipe for tomato chutney is so good, if you use it once on a hamburger you'll never touch ketchup again. It comes from an old New England family's maiden aunt, who jealously guarded the recipe during her lifetime. Every Christmas, she passed out jars of the chutney as gifts to eager recipients, who always begged for the recipe, but were always denied.

When she died, her relatives ransacked her kitchen looking for the recipe. One of them found it. I can no longer remember what favor I did in exchange for this recipe, but it was something onerous, like driving to the airport in rush hour on the Wednesday before Thanksgiving. I made a solemn promise never to reveal the source.

    3 pounds ripe tomatoes
    3 tart apples (green)
    2 cloves garlic
    1 cup raisins
    2 pieces (5-inch) of gingerroot, peeled and cut in half lengthwise
    3 cups brown sugar
    2 cups white vinegar
    1 tablespoon salt
    ¼ teaspoon cayenne

1. Put the tomatoes, apples, garlic, and raisins through a food chopper.
2. Combine these and all the other ingredients in a 3-quart pot and bring to a boil.
3. Simmer, stirring frequently, until the mixture is the consistency of apple butter.
4. Lift out the pieces of gingerroot.
5. Ladle into hot sterilized jars. Refrigerate.

YIELD: 3 to 4 pints

Valerian

BOTANICAL NAME: *Valeriana officinalis,* Valerianaceae.

COMMON NAME: Valerian.

DESCRIPTION: Hardy perennial.

> *Height:* To 4 feet.

> *Flowers:* Very pale pink, fragrant in June.

> *Leaves:* Large, handsome compound leaves.

HARVEST: Dig up the rhizomes at the end of the plant's second year of growth; remove fibrous roots before drying at temperatures below 200 degrees Fahrenheit.

CULTURE: Zones 3 to 10. Sun, moist soil. Valerian is suitable for growing in a container if kept moist. It is attractive to cats. Seeds are sometimes slow to start.

USE: An excellent sleep tonic is derived from the roots.

COMMENTS: Don't take valerian and drive; it causes drowsiness.

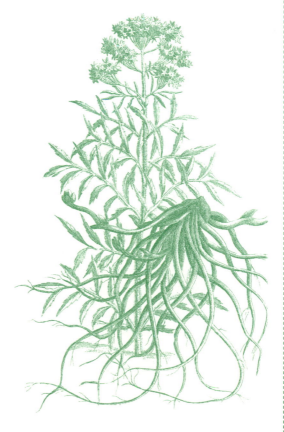

*V*alerian has a long history of use as a sedative. Administered to treat shell shock in World War I and for stress caused by air raids during World War II, valerian root is useful in the treatment of insomnia, hysteria, spasms, and anxiety. It is on the German Commission E's approved list for restlessness and sleeping disorders. Unless grossly overused (when it can cause headache and stupor), valerian has no aftereffects.

Whenever worry or a strange bed keeps me awake, I use a few drops of tincture of valerian in a cup of chamomile tea. It always works and it never makes me feel doped-up the next morning.

Because plants were not to be found locally, I grew valerian from seeds purchased by mail order. Started in mid-March, they weren't quick to germinate, as I remember, but neither were they so slow that I feared they were dead. By late May, stocky plants were ready to be transplanted into the garden.

In the wild in Britain and Europe, valerian is found in ditches and along rivers. While the plant thrives in rich, very moist soil, herbalists say that roots grown under drier conditions contain more of the essential oil. As I had no ditch or riverbank handy, I opted for a somewhat moister than average site, shaded by a picket fence. As soon as they were set into the ground the plants took off. I think that this had less to do with their site than with the fact that valerian, given any kind of decent situation, grows like the lusty wildflower it is.

Valerian turned out to be a beauty. The small plants eventually composed a tall, stately colony with elegantly cut leaves and pinky-white, sweetly scented flowers in June. I cut them for bouquets and found that the cutting stimulated the formation of more flowers.

In fall, it wasn't hard to dig up every other plant to harvest the roots, because the plants had more than filled their allotted spaces. It was comforting to know my own fresh, organically grown plants would be the source of next year's sleep tonic.

The spider-shaped roots did not live up to their reputation of smelling like moldering athletic socks. Rather, their aroma when freshly dug was medicinal. Only as they dried was there a hint of stale washcloth.

Because of its gentle effect, valerian is recommended for children suffering from hyperactivity. Before you dose a child, however, I'd advise seeing your pediatrician.

Knockout Decoction

Because it is the root of valerian that is the medicinal part, it takes more than simply steeping to obtain its benefits. A "decoction" is made by simmering the roots at a very low heat.

1 ounce fresh valerian root, chopped into small pieces
1 cup water

1. Combine valerian-root pieces and water in a saucepan.
2. Bring to a simmer and cover. Allow to simmer for 20 to 30 minutes.
3. Remove from heat and allow to cool for 20 to 30 minutes.
4. Strain and refrigerate.

NOTE: The decoction will keep for a week. For later use, freeze. Add a tablespoon to chamomile tea at bedtime.

List of Healing Plants by Use

Antioxidant, antiaging
Broccoli
Burdock
Carrot
Chive
Echinacea
Garlic
Ginseng
Goldenseal
Gotu kola
Mint
Nettle
Onion
Parsley
Purslane
Sage
Tomato

Bladder and kidney support
Asparagus
Blueberry
Burdock
Dandelion
Lovage
Purslane

Cough, cold and flu fighters
Anise
Chive
Echinacea
Elderberry

Elecampane
Garlic
Horehound
Hyssop
Mullein
Sage

Digestives
Anise
Caraway
Coriander
Dill
Elecampane (parasites)
Epazote (vermifuge)
Fennel seeds
Ginger
Goldenseal
Mint

Edible flowers
Anise
Bee balm
Caraway
Chive
Coriander
Dill
Elderberry
Garlic
Heartsease
Mexican mint
Rose

Headache fighters
Chamomile
Feverfew
Lemon balm

Lemongrass
Pumpkin
Onion

Heart and circulation aids
Carrot
Garlic
Onion
Parsley
Saffron
Tomato

Immune boosters
Burdock
Carrot
Echinacea
Elecampane
Ginseng
Goldenseal
Gotu kola
Purslane

Liver support
Milk thistle

Mood, dream, and sleep enhancers
Bee balm
Chamomile
Heartsease
Lavender
Lemon balm
Lemon verbena
Mugwort
Mullein
Saint-John's-wort
Valerian

Perennial border
Burnet
Chive
Echinacea
Elecampane
Lavender
Lemon balm
Lemongrass
Mint
Mullein
Rose
Rosemary
Saffron
Sunflower
Valerian

Phytoestrogens
Anise
Chaste tree
Fennel
Parsley
Strawberry

Prostate health
Pumpkin
Saw palmetto
Tomato

Shrubs
Bay
Blueberry
Chaste tree
Elderberry
Rose
Rosemary
Sage

Saw palmetto
Thyme

Supernutrients
Asparagus
Blueberry
Broccoli
Carrot
Chive
Lamb's-quarters
Parsley
Pepper
Purslane
Rose
Spinach
Strawberry
Sunflower seeds
Tomato

Tea
Bee balm
Chamomile
Coriander
Dill
Fennel
Feverfew
Lemon balm
Lemon verbena
Mint
Mullein
Nettle
Rose
Sage
Stevia
Thyme

Windowsill

Anise
Bay
Burnet
Caraway
Chervil
Chive
Cilantro
Dill
Epazote
Gotu kola
Lemongrass
Lemon verbena
Mexican mint
Parsley
Pepper
Rosemary
Stevia

Sources

SEEDS

The Banana Tree, Inc., 610-253-9589, *www.banana-tree.com*, catalog, Internet only.

The Cook's Garden, P.O. Box 535, Londonderry, VT 05148, 1-800-457-9703, fax 1-800-457-9705, *www.cooksgarden.com*.

Johnny's Selected Seeds, 1 Foss Hill Road, R.R. 1 Box 2580, Albion, ME 04910-9731, 207-437-4301, fax 800-437-4290, *www.johnnyseeds.com*.

Garden Medicinals and Culinaries, P.O. Box 320, Earlysville, VA 22936, 804-964-9113, fax 804-973-8717, *www.gardenmedicinals.com*, catalog $2.

The Gourmet Gardener, 8650 College Boulevard, Overland Park, KS 66210, 913-345-0490.

Prairie Moon Nursery, Route 3, Box 163, Winona, MN 55987, 507-452-1362, fax 507-454-5238, *www.prairiemoonnursery.com*.

Richters, 357 Highway 47, Goodwood, Ontario, Canada LOC 1A0, 905-640-6677, *www.richters.com*.

Seeds Blum, Idaho City Stage, Boise, ID 83706, 208-336-8264, catalog $3.

Seeds of Change, P.O. Box 15700, Santa Fe, NM 87506-5700, 1-888-762-7333, fax 1-888-329-4762, *www.seedsofchange.com*.

Shepherd's Garden Seeds, 30 Irene Street, Torrington, CT 06790-6627, 203-482-3638.

Southern Exposure Seed Exchange, P.O. Box 170, Earlysville, VA 22936.

Territorial Seed Company, P.O. Box 157, Cottage Grove, OR 97424-0061, 541-942-9547, fax 888-657-3131, *www.territorial-seed.com*.

The Thyme Garden Herb Seed Company, 20546 Alsea Highway, Alsea, OR 97324, 541-487-8671, *thymegarden@proaxis.com*, catalog $2.

Well-Sweep Herb Farm, 317 Mount Bethel Road, Port Murray, NJ 07865, 908-852-5390, catalog $2.

PLANTS

The Banana Tree, Inc., 610-253-9589, *www.banana-tree.com,* catalog, Internet only.

Carroll Gardens, 444 East Main Street, Westminster, MD 21157, 800-638-6334, catalog $2.

Goodwin Creek Gardens, P.O. Box 83, Williams, OR 97544, 541-846-7357, catalog $1.

Logee's Greenhouses, 141 North Street, Danielson, CT 06239, catalog $3.

Oregon Exotics, 1065 Messinger Road, Grants Pass, OR 97527, catalog $2.

Prairie Moon Nursery, Route 3, Box 163, Winona, MN 55987, 507-452-1362, fax 507-454-5238, *www.prairiemoonnursery.com.*

Richters, 357 Highway 47, Goodwood, Ontario, Canada LOC 1A0, 905-640-6677, *www.richters.com.*

Sandy Mush Herb Nursery, 316 Surrett Cove Road, Leicester, NC 28748-9622, catalog $6.

Southern Perennials & Herbs, 98 Bridges Road, Tylertown, MS 39667-9338, 800-774-0079, *www.s-p-h.com/.*

The Thyme Garden Herb Seed Company, 20546 Alsea Highway, Alsea, OR 97324, 541-487-8671, *thymegarden@proaxis.com,* catalog $2.

Prairie Moon Nursery, Route 3, Box 163, Winona, MN 55987-9515, 507-452-1362, fax 507-454-5238, *www.prairiemoonnursery.net.*

Well-Sweep Herb Farm, 317 Mount Bethel Road, Port Murray, NJ 07865, 908-852-5390, catalog $2.

BULK HERBS AND EQUIPMENT

Garden Medicinals and Culinaries, P.O. Box 320, Earlysville, VA 22936, 804-964-9113, fax 804-973-8717, *www.gardenmedicinals.com,* catalog $2.

Moonrise Herbs, 826 G Street, Suite H-H, Arcata, CA 95521, 800-603-8364, fax 707-822-0506, *www.moonrise.botanical.com,* catalog $1.

The Thyme Garden Herb Seed Company, 20546 Alsea Highway, Alsea, OR 97324, 541-487-8671, *thymegarden@proaxis.com,* catalog $2.

Dream pillow herbs and supplies:
Long Creek Herbs, P.O. Box 127, Blue Eye, MO 65611, 417-779-5450, *www.longcreekherbs.com,* catalog $2, refundable with first order.

Bibliography

American Herbal Pharmacopoeia. "St. John's Wort Monograph: The Herb for Depression." *HerbalGram* no. 40, Summer 1997.

Beckstrom-Sternberg, Stephen M., James A. Duke, and K. K. Wain. The Ethnobotany Database. *http://probe.halusda/gpv/8300/cgi-bin/browse/ethnobotdb.*

Blumenthal, Mark. "Echinacea Highlighted as Cold and Flu Remedy." *HerbalGram* no. 29, Spring/Summer 1993.

——. "Valerian: Nature's Sleep Aid." *Natural Healing & Alternative Medicine,* premiere issue, Rodale Press, Emmaus, PA, 1998.

Boxer, Arabella, and Philippa Back. *The Herb Book.* London: Octopus Books, 1980.

Broadhurst, C. Leigh. "Herbs for Energy." *Herbs for Health,* July/August 1997.

Brownell, Kelly. "The Pressure to Eat: Why We're Getting Fatter." *Nutrition Action Healthletter* 25, no. 6, July/August 1998.

Bubel, Nancy. "Mint Conditions." *Horticulture,* February 1985.

Cabrera, Chanchal. "Holistic Herbal Strategies for Enhanced Immune Function." Paper presented at the Fourth International Herb Symposium, Wheaton College, Norton, Massachusetts, June 26–28, 1998.

"Capsules: Newsbreaks in Herb Research." *Herbs for Health,* July/August 1997.

Carlsson, Sonja. *Die Hildegard von Bingen Küche.* Weyarn, Germany: Seehamer Verlag, 1999.

Castleman, Michael. *The Healing Herbs.* Emmaus, Pennsylvania: Rodale Press, 1991.

"Chemical Cuisine." *Nutrition Action Healthletter,* March 1999.

Colburn, Don. "New Antidepressants Lead to Falls Too." *Washington Post Health,* October 13, 1998.

The Complete German Commission E Monographs: Therapeutic Guide to Herbal Medicine. Edited by Mark Blumenthal et al. Austin, Texas: American Botanical Council; Boston, Massachusetts: Integrative Medicine Communications, 1998.

Dean, Carolyn, M.D. "The Best Herbs for Kids." *Great Life,* September 1998.

"Diet & Cancer, the Big Picture." *Nutrition Action Healthletter,* December 1998.

Dr. Duke's Phytochemical and Ethnobotanical Databases, *http://www.ars-grin.gov/duke/*

Duke, James A. *The Green Pharmacy*. Emmaus, Pennsylvania: Rodale Press, 1997.

———. "A Guide to Herbal Alternatives." *Herbs for Health,* November/December 1997.

The Ethnobotanical Research Directory, *http://hammock.ifas.ufl.edu/~michael/EB/.*

Grunwald, Joerg. "The European Phytomedicines: Market Figures, Trends, Analyses." *HerbalGram* no. 34, Summer 1995.

Halaska, M.; K. Raus; P. Beles; A. Maran; and K.G. Paithner. (Treatment of cyclical mastodynia using an extract of Vitex agnus castus: results of a double-blind comparison with a placebo; article in Czech). *Ceska Gynekol* 63, no. 5, October 1998.

Herbal Information Center, *http://www.kcweb.com/herb/gotu.htm.*

Herman, Robin. "Scientists Probe Eagerly for Causes of Aging." *Washington Post Health,* October 13, 1998.

Hobbs, Christopher. "Echinacea: A Literature Review." *HerbalGram* no. 30, Winter 1994.

———. "Milk Thistle Therapy." *Herbs for Health,* July/August 1997.

———. "St. John's Wort." *HerbalGram* no. 18/19, Fall 1998/Winter 1999.

———. *Vitex: the Women's Herb.* Interweave Press, 1990.

Horn, Vanessa. "Bathed in Fragrance." *Greatlife,* January 1999.

Huxtable, Ryan J. "The Intoxications of Elizabethan Drama." *Herbarist* no. 64, 1998.

Jacobson, Michael F.; Lisa Y. Lefferts; and Anne Witte Garland. *Safe Food: Eating Wisely in a Risky World.* Los Angeles: Living Planet Press, 1991.

Janiger, Oscar, M.D., and Philip Goldberg. *A Different Kind of Healing: Doctors Speak Candidly about Their Successes with Alternative Medicine.* New York: Jeremy P. Tarcher/Putnam, 1993.

Kapuler, A. M. "The Sunflowers: America's Golden Daisies of the Sun." *Peace Seeds Resource Journal,* 1997.

Khalsa, Karta Purkh Singh. "Heart-Healthy Hawthorne." *Great Life,* September 1998.

Lee, John R., M.D. *What Your Doctor May Not Tell You about Menopause: The Breakthrough Book on Natural Progesterone.* New York: Warner Books, 1996.

Liebster, Gunther. *Berry Gardening.* Translated by Carole Ottesen. New York: Macmillan, 1986.

Luna, Rose. "Myth, Legend, and Magic: Sacred Herbs of Summer." Paper presented at the Fourth International Herb Symposium, Wheaton College, Norton, Massachusetts, June 26–28, 1998.

Mars, Brigitte. "Herbal Teas Health in a Cup." *Herbs for Health,* November/December 1997.

McCaleb, Rob. "Anti-cancer Effects of Gotu Kola," *HerbalGram* no. 36, Spring 1996.

———. "Lavender Oil Aromatherapy." *HerbalGram* no. 33, Spring 1995.

———. "New World Medicinal Plants." *HerbalGram* no. 27, Summer 1992.

———. "Research Reviews." *HerbalGram* no. 33, Spring, 1995.

———. "St. John's Wort Treats Depression." *HerbalGram* no. 33, Spring 1995.

McCaleb, Rob, and Don Brown. "Melissa: Relief for Herpes Sufferers." *Herbal-Gram* no. 34, Summer 1995.

McCaleb, Rob, and Ginger Webb. "Echinacea Clinical Studies Reviewed." *HerbalGram* no. 37, Summer 1996.

———. "Peppermint Oil and Irritable Bowel Syndrome." *HerbalGram* no. 37, Summer 1996.

Mint: Indiana Celebrates Leadership in Supplying Mint to the World. Marcia Pearson Press, 1996.

Meyerowitz, Steve. *Sprouts, the Miracle Food.* Great Barrington, Massachusetts: Sprout House, 1997.

Myers, Charles, M.D. "Should Diet Be Used to Help Treat Incurable Cancers? Yes." *Washington Post Health,* February 24, 1998.

Murray, Frank. "The Leading Edge." *Great Life,* September 1988.

Murray, Michael T., M.D. "Enteric-Coated Peppermint Oil for Irritable Bowel Syndrome." *Ask the Doctor,* Vital Communications, 1998.

———. "For Maximum Benefits Use Fresh Garlic Preparations." *Ask the Doctor,* Vital Communications, 1998.

———. "St. John's Wort Extract." *Ask the Doctor,* Vital Communications, 1997.

———. "Saw Palmetto Extract: Nature's Answer to Prostate Enlargement." *Ask the Doctor,* Vital Communications, 1998.

Native American Ethnobotany Database, *www.umd.umich.edu/cgi-bin/herb.*

Okie, Susan, "Information Gap on Herbal Products." *Washington Post Health,* September 29, 1998.

"Potent Blueberries." *Herbs for Health,* July/August 1997.

Potter, John D. "Diet and Cancer." *Nutrition Action,* December 1998.

Prevention Magazine Health Books Editors. *The Complete Book of Natural & Medicinal Cures.* Emmaus, Pennsylvania: Rodale Press, 1994.

"Research Reviews." *HerbalGram* no. 39, Spring 1997.

Rossbach, Sarah. *Feng Shui: The Chinese Art of Placement.* New York: Dutton, 1983.

Schardt, David. "Herbs for Nerves." *Nutrition Action Healthletter,* October 1998.

———. "Magnesium." *Nutrition Action Healthletter,* December 1998.

Shandler, Nina. *Estrogen the Natural Way: Over 250 Easy and Delicious Recipes for Menopause.* New York: Villard Books, 1997.

Smith, Ed. "Optimizing Health & Longevity with Anti-Aging and Adaptogenic Herbs." Paper presented at the Fourth International Herb Symposium, Wheaton College, Norton, Massachusetts, June 26–28, 1998.

———. "Sexy Herbs." Paper presented at the Fourth International Herb Symposium, Wheaton College, Norton, Massachusetts, June 26–28, 1998.

Squires, Sally. "Americans Eat Better but Not Quite Well." *Washington Post Health,* October 6, 1998.

———. "Researchers Weigh Tea's Health Benefits." *Washington Post Health,* October 6, 1998.

"Sweet Stevia." *Avant Gardener* 3, no. 5, May 1998.

Thompson, William A. R., M.D., ed. *Medicines from the Earth: A Guide to Healing Plants.* Revised by Richard Evans Schultes. San Francisco: Alfred Van Der Marck Editions, dist. by Harper & Row, 1983.

Thornton, Linda. "The Ethics of Wildcrafting." *Herb Quarterly,* Fall 1998.

Tucker, Arthur O. "The Truth about Mints." *Herb Companion,* August/September 1992.

———. "Growing Lavender." *Herbarist* no. 64, 1998.

Tyler, Varro E. "Combine with Care." *Sarasota Herald Tribune,* September 9, 1998.

———. *Herbs of Choice: The Therapeutic Use of Phylomedicinals.* New York: Pharmaceutical Products Press, 1994.

———. *The Honest Herbal: A Sensible Guide to the Use of Herbs and Related Remedies.* New York: Pharmaceutical Products Press, 1993.

Wang, D.V.C. "Feverfew Fever." *HerbalGram* no. 29, Spring/Summer 1993.

Warner, Charles Dudley. "In Praise of Dirt." In *The Gardener's World,* edited by Joseph Wood Krutch. New York: G. P. Putnam's Sons, 1959.

Webb, Densie. "Veggies Come Clean." *Greatlife,* January 1999.

Webb, Ginger. "Valerian Safety Confirmed in Overdose." *HerbalGram* no. 36, Spring 1996.

Weil, Andrew. "Hormone Mimics: An Emerging Threat." *Self Healing,* February 1999.

———. "New Findings in Natural Medicine." *Self Healing,* February 1999.

———. "New Findings in Natural Medicine." *Self Healing,* April 1999.

Wydra, Nancilee. *Feng Shui in the Garden.* Chicago: Contemporary Books, 1997.

Index

A. Brockie Stevenson's Dilled, Chilled
    Carrot Soup, 42–43
Accidental Curried Pumpkin Soup,
    196–197
Adams, James, 134, 135, 147
Aghevli, Joan, 188, 216
Aloe *(Aloe vera)*, 3–4
Angier, Bradford, 130, 242
Anise *(Pimpinella anisum)*, 5–6, 255, 256,
    258, 260
    aniseed bread, 7
    biscotti, 7–8
Applesauce, Sage, 222
Asparagus *(Asparagus officinalis)*, 9–10,
    255, 259
    with Spring Greens, 12
    Sue Watterson's Asparagus and Ham
        Strudel, 11–12

Barclay, Gwen, 83
Bay *(Laurus nobilis)*, 13–14, 258, 260
    Bouquet Garni, 15
    Hopping John Cassoulet, 14–16
Bee Balm *(Monarda didyma)*, 17–19, 256,
    257, 259
    Crab Cakes with, 20–21
    Pasta with—Basil Pesto, 19–20
    Vinaigrette, 19
Biscotti, Anise, 7–8
Black Bean–Cornmeal Muffins with
    Cilantro, 60–61
Blueberry *(Vaccinium corymbosum)*, 22–23,
    255, 258, 259
    Russian Blueberry and Raspberry
        Pudding Nora, 24
Bouquet Garni, 15
Bread
    Aniseed, 7
    Pumpkin, with Pepitas, 198

Bread Salad with Garden Thinnings,
    139–140
Broccoli *(Brassica oleracea)*, 25–27, 255,
    259
    growing sprouts, 27–28
    marinated, 28
    Sue Watterson's Dim Sum Broccoli,
        28–29
Burdock *(Arctium lappa)*, 30–31, 255,
    257
    Soup, 32
Burgess, Barbara, 193
Burnet *(Sanguisorba minor)*, 33–34, 258,
    260
    Soothing Burnet Wash, 35
    Vinegar, 35
Butters
    Carrots with Rosemary, 42
    Epazote, 86
    Mexican Mint and Watercress,
        157–158
    Parsley, 186–187
    Shallot, 183

Cabrera, Chanchal, 234
Caraway *(Carum carvi)*, 36–37, 256, 260
    Caraway Crackers, 38
    preparing seeds, 37
    Thyme Garden's Harissa, 39
Carrot *(Daucus carota)*, 40–41, 255, 257,
    259
    A. Brockie Stevenson's Dilled, Chilled
        Carrot Soup, 42–43
    with Rosemary Butter, 42
Chamomile *(Matricaria recutita)*, 44–46,
    256, 257, 259
    harvesting flowers for tea, 46–47
    Sleep Tea, 47
    Under-Eye Oil, 47–48

Chaste Tree *(Vitex agnus-castus)*, 49–50, 258
  Hormone-Balance Tincture, 51
Chervil *(Anthriscus cerefolium)*, 52–53, 260
  Fines Herbes Oil, 53
Chicken
  Hot and Spicy Chicken Soup, 192
  Hyssop Chicken for Sadnesse, 126–127
  Mexican Mint Picnic, 159–160
Chickpea–Lamb's-quarters Curry, 132
Chili, Cold Season Rose Hip, 206–207
Chive *(Allium schoenoprasum)*, 54–55, 255, 256, 258–260
  Salmon "Scallopini" with Chive Cream, 56
  Vinaigrette, 55–56
Chunky Gazpacho with Lemon Balm, 104–105
Chutney, X's Aunt's Tomato, 250
Cilantro *(see* Coriander [*Coriandum sativum*])
Coffee Cake, Rose Hip, 205–206
Cold Lovage-Potato Soup, 154–155
Complete Book of Natural & Medicinal Cures, The, 185
Cooper, Mary, 213
Cordial
  Elderberry, 76–77
  Elecampane, 80–81
Coriander *(Coriandum sativum)*, 57–58, 256, 259, 260
  Black Bean–Cornmeal Muffins with Cilantro, 60–61
  Curried Lentils, 59–60
  Curry in a Hurry, 58–59
  Thyme Garden's Harissa, 39
Country Housewife's Handbook, The, 76
Crab Cakes with Bee Balm, 20–21
Crackers, Caraway, 38
Crème Brûlée
  Lavender, 136–137
  Mellow Yellow, 150
Crêpes, Lamb's-quarters, 130–132
Cumin, Thyme Garden's Harissa, 39

Curry
  Accidental Curried Pumpkin Soup, 196–197
  Curry in a Hurry, 58–59
  Lamb's-quarters–Chickpea, 132
  Lentils, 59–60
Curry in a Hurry, 58–59

Dandelion *(Taraxacum officinale)*, 62–64, 255
  Classic Greens, 66–67
  Dandelion Root Tea, 64
  Lasagna with Shiitakes, 64–65
  roasting roots, 65
Desserts *(see also* Ice Cream)
  Gingered Pear Tart, 110
  Hyssop-Peach Tart, 128
  Jan's Peppermint Sorbet, 166–167
  Lavender Crème Brûlée, 136–137
  Lavender Ice Cream, 135
  Mary Cooper's Rosemary Cookies, 213
  Mellow Yellow Crème Brûlée, 150
  The Only Good Fruitcake, 207–208
  Rose Hip Coffee Cake, 205–206
  Rosemary Shortbread, 212
  Russian Blueberry and Raspberry Pudding Nora, 24
  Sue's Strawberry Dessert Salad, 238
Dill *(Anethum graveolens)*, 68–69, 256, 259, 260
  Hummus, 70–71
  salt method for preserving, 69
  Tomato, Red Onion, and Dill Salad Bella Luna, 70
Dilled, Chilled Carrot Soup, 42–43
Dim Sum Broccoli, 28–29
Dionot, François, 56, 103, 187
Dioscorides, 97, 126
Duke, James, 4, 87, 97, 113, 120, 133, 200, 220, 237
Durough, Steve, 249–250

Echinacea *(Echinacea purpurea)*, 72–74, 255, 257, 258
  Echinacea Root Tea, 74
  preparing roots for storage, 74

Eggs Benedict on Smoked Turkey Hash, 159

Elderberry *(Sambucus canadensis)*, 75–76, 256, 258
  Cordial (nonalcoholic), 76–77
  drying flowers, 77
  Elderberry Flowers Tempura, 77–78

Elecampane *(Inula helenium)*, 79–80, 256–258
  Cordial, 80–81

Enchanted Broccoli Forest, The (Katzen), 168

Epazote *(Chenopodium ambroisiodes)*, 82–83, 256, 260
  -Artemisia Room Freshener, 85–86
  Butter, 86
  Juan's Sopa de Albóndiga (Meatball Soup), 84
  Sopa de Setas (Wild Mushroom Soup), 85

Erdman, John, 42

Estrogen the Natural Way (Shandler), 38

Fava beans *(Vicia faba)*, 87–88
  Nora's Succotash, 88–89

Feasting Free on Wild Edibles (Angier), 242

Fennel *(Foeniculum vulgare)*, 90–92, 256, 258, 259
  Fennel, Orange, and Cabbage Salad, 93–94
  Herbes de Provence, 93
  Terry Pogue's Fennel and Apple Salad, 94–95

Feverfew *(Tanacetum parthenium)*, 96–97, 256, 259
  -Cucumber Sandwich, 98
  Tea, 98

Fines Herbes Oil, 53

Fish
  Red Snapper Fillet with Lemongrass, 147
  Salmon "Scallopini" with Chive Cream, 56

François Dionot's Cold Fresh Herb Soup, 187–188

Fried Green Tomatoes à la Steve Durough, 249–250

Galen, 123

Gargle, Sage, 222

Garlic *(Allium sativum)*, 99–102, 255, 256, 257
  Chunky Gazpacho with Lemon Balm, 104–105
  flower stalks, 104
  Roasted Garlic and Eggplant Soup, 103
  Roasted Garlic Grits, 105–106
  Rosettes, 104

German Commission E, 4, 6, 10, 37, 50, 58, 63, 69, 74, 76, 108, 113, 120, 123, 133, 139, 174, 185, 202, 224, 227, 245

Ginger *(Zingiber officinale)*, 107–109, 256
  as gas reliever, 109
  Gingered Pear Tart, 110
  Pommes de Marie-Eve, 109
  -Thyme Dressing, 247

Ginseng *(Panax quinquefolius)*, 111–113, 255, 257

Goldenseal *(Hydrastis canadensis)*, 114–116, 255, 256, 257

Gotu Kola *(Centella asiatica)*, 117–118, 255, 257, 260
  Calm and Centered Tea, 118

Grilled Marinated Vegetables, 193–194

Grits, Roasted Garlic, 105–106

Heartsease *(Viola tricolor)*, 119–120, 256, 257
  Salad, 121

Herbes de Provence, 93

Herb Society of Central Indiana, 167

Hildegard von Bingen, 123, 126

Hill, Madelene, 83

Hobbs, Christopher, 50

Hollandaise, Mexican mint, 158

Homemade Zahtar, 246–247

Hopping John Cassoulet, 14–16

Horehound *(Marrubium vulgare)*, 122–123, 256
  Syrup, 123–124
Hormone-Balance Tincture, 51
Hummus, Dill, 70–71
Hunter-Gatherer Breakfast Mix, 243–244
Hussein, Rabia, 58–59
Hyssop *(Hyssopus officinalis)*, 125–126, 256
  Hyssop Chicken for Sadnesse, 126–127
  -Peach Tart, 128

Ice Cream
  Joan Aghevli's Saffron, 216
  Lavender, 135
Iced Coffee, Mint, 167
Indiana Cold Mint Pea Salad, 168–169

Jan Midgley's Classic Greens, 66–67
Jan Midgley's Peppermint Sorbet, 166–167
Jerusalem artichoke *(Helianthus tuberosus)*, 243
Joan Aghevli's Mast-O-Khiar, 208
Joan Aghevli's Persian Rice, 188–189
Joan Aghevli's Saffron Ice Cream, 216
Johnny-jump-up (*see* Heartsease [*Viola tricolor*])
Johnny's Selected Seeds, 27

Kamut with Parsley and Onion Greens, 186
Katzen, Mollie, 168
Kennedy, Diana, 83
Klamath weed (*see* Saint-John's-wort [*Hypericum perforatum*])
Knockout Decoction, 253

Lamb's-quarters *(Chenopodium album)*, 129–130, 259
  –Chickpea Curry, 132
  Crêpes, 130–132
Lamb with a Peppermint Crust, 168
Lancet, The, 97, 108

Lavender *(Lavandula angustifolia)*, 133–135, 257, 258
  Crème Brûlée, 136–137
  Ice Cream, 135
  Spritzer, 137
  Sugar, 137
Lemon Balm *(Melissa officinalis)*, 138–139, 257–259
  Bread Salad with Garden Thinnings, 139–140
  Chunky Gazpacho with Lemon Balm, 104–105
  Dressing, 140–141
Lemongrass *(Cymbopogon citratus)*, 142–144, 257, 258, 260
  Bows, 145
  Braid for Tea, 144
  Red Snapper Fillet with, 147
  Romy's Tom Khar, 146–147
  Soup Asia Nora, 144–146
Lemon Verbena *(Aloysia triphylla)*, 148–149, 257, 259, 260
  drying, 149
  Mellow Yellow Crème Brûlée, 150
  Sugar, 151
Lentils, Curried, 59–60
Long, Jim, 172
Long Creek Herbs Sleep Pillow, 172
Lovage *(Levisticum officinale)*, 152–153, 255
  Cold Lovage-Potato Soup, 154–155
  and Tomatoes, 153–154

MacQueen, Marilyn, 193
Making Herbal Dream Pillows (Long), 172
Malcolm, Christine, 134
Mancini, Romy, 146
Mary Cooper's Rosemary Cookies, 213
Mast-O-Khiar, 208
Mexican Mint *(Tagetes lucida)*, 156–157, 256, 260
  Dressing, 160
  Eggs Benedict on Smoked Turkey Hash, 159
  Hollandaise, 158

Picnic Chicken, 159–160
and Watercress Butter, 157–158
Meyerowitz, Steve, 27
Midgley, Jan, 66, 166
Milk Thistle *(Silybum marianum)*,
161–163, 257
Morning-After Tonic, 163
Mint *(Mentha* spp.), 164–166, 255, 256,
258, 259
forcing for winter use, 166
Iced Coffee, 167
Indiana Cold Mint Pea Salad,
168–169
Jan Midgley's Peppermint Sorbet,
166–167
Lamb with a Peppermint Crust, 168
Mrs. Adams's Salt Method for Preserving
Dill, 69
Morning-After Milk Thistle Tonic, 163
Muffins, Black Bean–Cornmeal Muffins
with Cilantro, 60–61
Mugwort *(Artemisia vulgaris)*, 170–172,
257
Long Creek Herbs Sleep Pillow, 172
Mullein *(Verbascum thapsus)*, 173–174,
256–259
Serene Slumber Tea, 174–175
Murray, Michael T., 227

Nettle *(Urtica dioica)*, 176–178, 255, 259
fertilizer, 179
-Flecked Parsnips and Turnips,
178–179
Soup, 179–180
Tea, 178
Nora's Fava Bean Succotash, 88–89
Nora's Lemongrass Soup Asia, 144–146
Nora's Russian Blueberry and Raspberry
Pudding, 24
Nora's Saffron Risotto with Shrimp and
Peas, 217–218

Oatcakes, Sage, 221
Oil, Saint-John's-wort, 225
Onion *(Allium* spp.), 181–183, 255,
257

curing, 183
Shallot Butter, 183
The Only Good Fruitcake, 207–208

Parkinson, John, 97
Parsley *(Petroselinum crispum* var.
neoplitanum), 184–185, 255,
257–260
Butter, 186–187
François Dionot's Cold Fresh Herb
Soup, 187–188
Joan Aghevli's Persian Rice, 188–189
Kamut with Parsley and Onion
Greens, 186
Parsnips and Turnips, Nettle-Flecked,
178–179
Pasta
with Bee Balm–Basil Pesto, 19–20
Dandelion Lasagna with Shiitakes,
64–65
Pepper *(Capsicum* spp.), 190–192, 259,
260
Grilled Marinated Vegetables,
193–194
Hot and Spicy Chicken Soup, 192
Queensdale Spicy Pepper Marinade,
193
Pfeifer, Horst, 70
Pogue, Terry, 94, 205
Pommes de Marie-Eve, 109
Pouillon, Nora, 144, 154, 217
Pratt, Barbara, 93
Prevention Magazine Health Books,
185
Pumpkin *(Cucurbita pepo)*, 195–196, 257,
258
Accidental Curried Pumpkin Soup,
196–197
Bread with Pepitas, 198
storing, 196
Purslane *(Portulaca oleracea sativa)*,
199–200, 255, 257, 259
Stir-Fry Soup, 201

Queensdale Spicy Pepper Marinade,
193

Riddell, Neil, 109
Rieman, Margo, 14
Roasted Garlic Grits, 105–106
Romy's Tom Khar, 146–147
Rose (*Rosa* spp.), 202–203, 256, 258, 259
  Cold Season Rose Hip Chili, 206–207
  Joan's Mast-O-Khiar, 208
  The Only Good Fruitcake, 207–208
  Rose Hip Coffee Cake, 205–206
  Rose Hip Purée, 204
  Rose Water, 209
  types of, 203–204
Rosemary *(Rosmarinus officinalis)*, 210–211, 258, 260
  Butter with Carrots, 42
  Mary Cooper's Rosemary Cookies, 213
  Shortbread, 212
Russian Blueberry and Raspberry Pudding Nora, 24

Saffron *(Crocus sativus)*, 214–215, 257, 258
  Joan Aghevli's Saffron Ice Cream, 216
  Nora's Saffron Risotto with Shrimp and Peas, 217–218
  using, 216
Sage *(Salvia officinalis)*, 219–221, 255, 256, 259
  Applesauce, 222
  Gargle, 222
  Oatcakes, 221
  Tea, 220–221
Saint-John's-wort *(Hypericum perforatum)*, 223–224, 257
  Oil, 225
Salad dressings
  Chive Vinaigrette, 55–56
  Lemon Balm, 140–141
  Mexican Mint, 160
  Monarda Vinaigrette, 19
  Thyme-Ginger Dressing, 247

Salads
  Bread Salad with Garden Thinnings, 139–140
  Fennel, Orange, and Cabbage Salad, 93–94
  Heartsease, 121
  Indiana Cold Mint Pea Salad, 168–169
  Jan Midgley's Classic Greens, 66–67
  Joan's Mast-O-Khiar, 208
  Terry Pogue's Fennel and Apple Salad, 94–95
  Tomato, Red Onion, and Dill Salad Bella Luna, 70
Salmon "Scallopini" with Chive Cream, 56
Sands, Stephen, 136
Sandwiches, Feverfew-Cucumber, 98
Saw Palmetto *(Serenoa repens)*, 226–227, 258, 259
  Prostate-Preserving Tonic, 228
Shallots (*see* Onion [*Allium* spp.])
Shandler, Nina, 38
Sharif, Linda, 246
Shiitake Creamed Spinach, 230–231
Shimizu, Holly, 134
Shortbread, Rosemary, 212
Sleep Pillow, 172
Sleep Tea, 47
Smith, Ed, 113
Soups
  A. Brockie Stevenson's Dilled, Chilled Carrot, 42–43
  Accidental Curried Pumpkin, 196–197
  Burdock, 32
  Chunky Gazpacho with Lemon Balm, 104–105
  Cold Lovage-Potato, 154–155
  François Dionot's Cold Fresh Herb, 187–188
  Hot and Spicy Chicken, 192
  Juan's Sopa de Albóndiga (Meatball Soup), 84
  Lemongrass Asia Nora, 144–146
  Nettle, 179–180
  Roasted Garlic and Eggplant, 103

Sopa de Setas (Wild Mushroom
   Soup), 85
Stir-Fry Soup with Purslane, 201
Southern Herb Growing (Hill and Barclay),
   83
Spinach *(Spinacia oleracea)*, 229–230, 259
   and Ham Strudel, 231–232
   Shiitake Creamed Spinach, 230–231
Spritzer, Lavender, 137
Sprouts, the Miracle Food (Meyerowitz), 27
Stevenson, A. Brockie, 42
Stevia *(Stevia rebaudiana)*, 233–235, 259,
   260
   Syrup, 235
Strawberry *(Fragaria* spp.), 236–237,
   258, 259
   Leaf Tea, 237–238
   Sue Watterson's Strawberry Dessert
      Salad, 238
Strudel
   Asparagus and Ham, 11–12
   Spinach and Ham, 231–232
Sue Watterson's Asparagus and Ham
   Strudel, 11–12
Sue Watterson's Dim Sum Broccoli,
   28–29
Sue Watterson's Strawberry Dessert
   Salad, 238
Sugar
   Lavender, 137
   Lemon Verbena, 151
Sumac *(Rhus* spp.), 239–240
   Sumac Drink and Sorbet, 240
Sunflower *(Helianthus annuus)*, 241–242,
   258, 259
   curing seeds, 242
   Hunter-Gatherer Breakfast Mix,
      243–244
   Jerusalem artichoke, 243
Syrup
   Horehound, 123–124
   Stevia, 235

Talley, Kris, 76
Teas
   Bee Balm, 19

Calm and Centered (Gotu Kola),
   118
Dandelion Root, 64
Echinacea Root, 74
Feverfew, 98
Lemon Balm, 139
Lemongrass, 144
Lemon Verbena, 148, 149
Mint, 164, 166
Nettle, 178
Rose, 202
Sage, 220–221
Serene Slumber Tea (Mullein),
   174–175
Sleep Tea (Chamomile), 47
Strawberry Leaf, 237–238
Thyme, 246
Territorial Seed Company, 242
Terry Pogue's Fennel and Apple Salad,
   94–95
Thornton, Linda, 227
Thyme *(Thymus* spp.), 245–246, 259
   -Ginger Dressing, 247
   Homemade Zahtar, 246–247
   Tea, 246
   types of, 246
Thyme Garden Herb Seed Company
   Harissa, 39
Tomato *(Lycopersicon lycopersicum)*,
   248–249, 255, 257–259
   Fried Green Tomatoes à la Steve
      Durough, 249–250
   and Lovage, 153–154
   and Red Onion, and Dill Salad, 70
   X's Aunt's Tomato Chutney, 250
Tucker, Arthur O., 165
Twelve Company Dinners (Rieman), 14
Tyler, Varro E., 123, 162

Under-Eye Oil, Chamomile, 47–48

Valerian *(Valeriana officinalis)*, 251–252,
   257, 258
   Knockout Decoction, 253
Vinaigrette
   Bee Balm, 19

Vinaigrette *(cont.)*
 Chive, 55–56
 Lemon Balm, 140–141
Vinegar, Burnet, 35

Watterson, Sue, 7, 11, 28, 231,
 238

White horehound (*see* Horehound
 [*Marrubium vulgare*])

X's Aunt's Tomato Chutney, 250

Zahtar, Homemade, 246–247
Zuchowicz, Nicki, 85

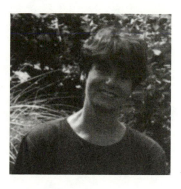

ABOUT THE AUTHOR

CAROLE OTTESEN is an organic gardener and author of *The New American Garden, Ornamental Grasses,* and *The Native Plant Primer.* She lectures widely and is well known for her trendsetting gardening sensibilities. She lives in Potomac, Maryland.